ECSI Emergency Care and Safety Institute

First Aid and CPR Essentials

Fifth Edition

Alton Thygerson, Ed.D.
Medical Writer

Benjamin Gulli, MD
Medical Editor

Jon R. Krohmer, MD, FACEP
Medical Editor

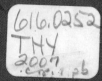

American College of
Emergency Physicians®
ADVANCING EMERGENCY CARE

JONES AND BARTLETT PUBLISHERS
Sudbury, Massachusetts
BOSTON   TORONTO   LONDON   SINGAPORE

Jones and Bartlett Publishers

World Headquarters
40 Tall Pine Drive
Sudbury, MA 01776
info@jbpub.com
www.ECSInstitute.org

Jones and Bartlett Publishers Canada
6339 Ormindale Way
Mississauga, Ontario L5V 1J2
Canada

Jones and Bartlett Publishers International
Barb House, Barb Mews
London W6 7PA
United Kingdom

Jones and Bartlett's books and products are available through most bookstores and online booksellers. To contact Jones and Bartlett Publishers directly, call 800-832-0034, fax 978-443-8000, or visit our website www.jbpub.com.

Substantial discounts on bulk quantities of Jones and Bartlett's publications are available to corporations, professional associations, and other qualified organizations. For details and specific discount information, contact the special sales department at Jones and Bartlett via the above contact information or send an email to specialsales@jbpub.com.

Production Credits
Chief Executive Officer: Clayton E. Jones
Chief Operating Officer: Donald W. Jones, Jr.
President, Higher Education and Professional Publishing: Robert W. Holland, Jr.
V.P., Sales and Marketing: William J. Kane
V.P., Production and Design: Anne Spencer
V.P., Manufacturing and Inventory Control: Therese Connell
Publisher: Lawrence Newell
Publisher, Public Safety Group: Kimberly Brophy
Acquisitions Editor: Christine Emerton
Editor: Jennifer S. Kling

American Academy of Orthopaedic Surgeons

Associate Managing Editor: Amanda Green
Production Supervisor: Jenny L. Corriveau
Associate Photo Researcher: Christine McKeen
Director of Marketing: Alisha Weisman
Interior Design: Anne Spencer
Cover Design: Kristin E. Ohlin
Cover Image: © Jones and Bartlett Publishers. Photographed by Kimberly Potvin.
Composition: Shepherd, Inc.
Text Printing and Binding: Courier Kendallville
Cover Printing: Courier Kendallville

The first aid and CPR procedures in this book are based on the most current recommendations of responsible medical sources. The American Academy of Orthopaedic Surgeons and the Publisher, however, make no guarantee as to, and assume no responsibility for, the correctness, sufficiency, or completeness of such information or recommendations. Other or additional safety measures may be required under particular circumstances.

Reviewed by the American College of Emergency Physicians

The American College of Emergency Physicians (ACEP) makes every effort to ensure that its product and program reviewers are knowledgeable content experts and recognized authorities in their fields. Readers are nevertheless advised that the statements and opinions expressed in this publication are provided as guidelines and should not be construed as College policy unless specifically referred to as such. The College disclaims any liability or responsibility for the consequences of any actions taken in reliance on those statements or opinions. The materials contained herein are not intended to establish policy, procedure, or a standard of care. To contact ACEP write to: PO Box 619911, Dallas, TX 75261-9911; call toll-free 800-798-1822, touch 6, or 972-550-0911.

Library of Congress Cataloging-in-Publication Data

ISBN-13: 978-0-7637-4226-3
ISBN-10: 0-7637-4226-0

6048

Additional photographic and illustration credits appear on page 205, which constitutes a continuation of the copyright page.

Printed in the United States of America
10 09 08 07 06   10 9 8 7 6 5 4 3 2 1

contents

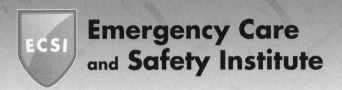

welcome

Welcome to the Emergency Care and Safety Institute

Welcome to the Emergency Care and Safety Institute (ECSI), brought to you by the American Academy of Orthopaedic Surgeons (AAOS) and the American College of Emergency Physicians (ACEP).

The ECSI is an educational organization created for the purpose of delivering the highest quality training to laypersons and professionals in the areas of First Aid, CPR, AED, Bloodborne Pathogens, and related safety and health fields.

Two of the most respected names in injury, illness, and emergency medical care—AAOS and ACEP—have approved the content of our training materials.

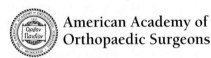

American Academy of Orthopaedic Surgeons

About the AAOS

The AAOS provides education and practice management services for orthopaedic surgeons and allied health professionals. The AAOS also serves as an advocate for improved patient care and informs the public about the science of orthopaedics. Founded in 1933, the not-for-profit AAOS has grown from a small organization serving less than 500 members to the world's largest medical association of musculoskeletal specialists. The AAOS now serves about 24,000 members internationally.

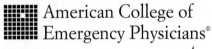

American College of Emergency Physicians®

ADVANCING EMERGENCY CARE

About ACEP

ACEP was founded in 1968 and is the world's oldest and largest emergency medicine specialty organization. Today it represents more than 23,000 members and is the emergency medicine specialty society recognized as the acknowledged leader in emergency medicine.

ECSI Course Catalog

Individuals seeking training in ECSI subjects can choose from among various online and offline course offerings. The following courses are available through the ECSI:

First Aid, CPR, and AED Standard

CPR and AED

Professional Rescuer CPR

First Aid

Wilderness First Aid

Bloodborne Pathogens

First Responder

First Aid and CPR Online

First Aid Online

Adult CPR Online

Adult and Pediatric CPR Online

Professional Rescuer CPR Online

AED Online

Adult CPR and AED Online

Bloodborne Pathogens Online

The ECSI offers a wide range of textbooks, instructor and student support materials, and interactive technology, including online courses. Every ECSI textbook is the center of an integrated teaching and learning system that offers instructor, student, and technology resources to better support instructors and prepare students. The instructor supplements provide practical hands-on, time-saving tools like PowerPoint presentations, DVDs, and web-based distance learning resources. The student supplements are designed to help students retain the most important information and to assist them in preparing for exams. And, a key component to the teaching and learning systems are technology resources that provide interactive exercises and simulations to help students become great emergency responders.

Documents attesting to the ECSI's recognitions of satisfactory course completion will be issued to those who successfully meet the course objectives and criteria for passing the course. Written acknowledgement of a participant's successful course completion is provided in the form of a Course Completion Card, issued by the ECSI.

Visit www.ECSInstitute.org today!

resource preview

This textbook is part of the First Aid and CPR program with features that will reinforce and expand on the essential information.

Features include:

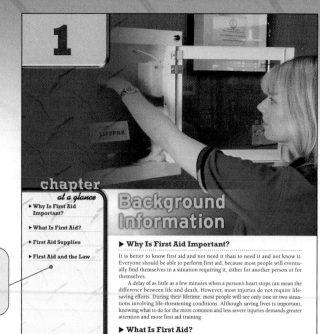

Chapter at a Glance
Guide students through the topics covered in that chapter.

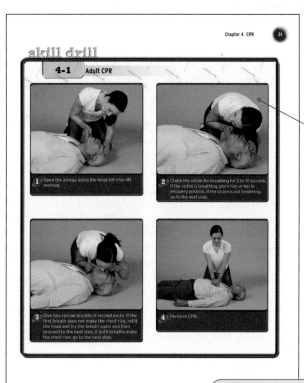

Skill Drills
Provide step-by-step explanations and visual summaries of important skills for first aiders.

Caution Boxes
Emphasize crucial actions that first aiders should or should not take while administering treatment.

FYI Boxes
Include valuable information related to the injuries or illnesses discussed in that section, including prevention tips and risk factors.

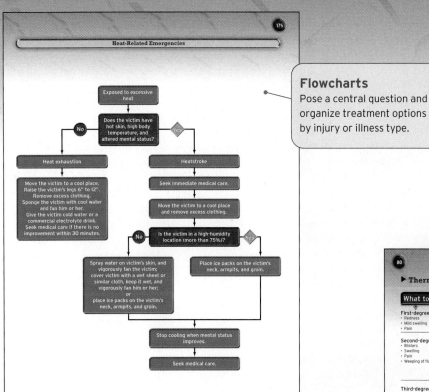

Flowcharts

Pose a central question and organize treatment options by injury or illness type.

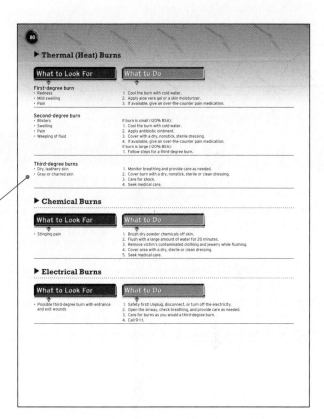

Decision Tables

Provide a concise summary of what signs first aiders should look for and what treatment steps they should take.

Prep Kit

End-of-chapter activities reinforce important concepts and improve students' comprehension.

Ready for Review: Provide a quick review of basic concepts.

Vital Vocabulary: A list of the key terms and definitions are provided for each chapter.

Assessment in Action: A brief case study is followed by critical thinking questions that allow students to apply what they've learned.

Check Your Knowledge: The questions quiz students on the chapter's core concepts.

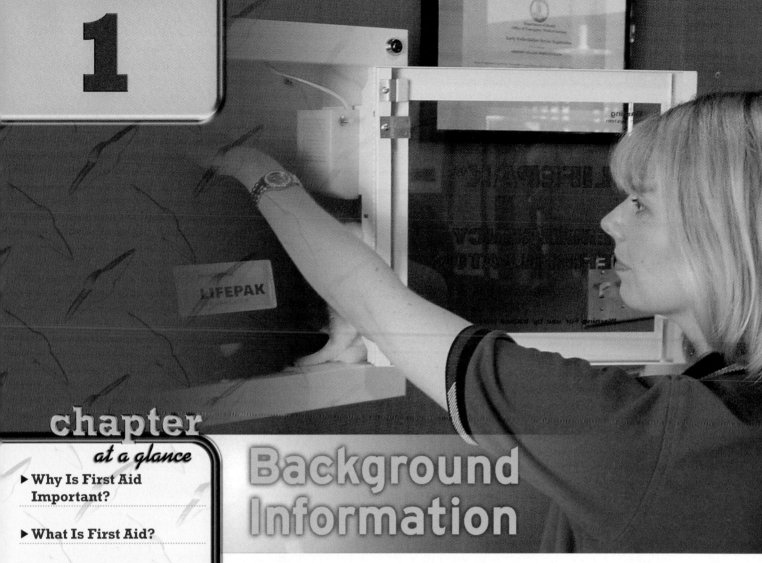

chapter
at a glance

Background Information

▶ Why Is First Aid Important?

It is better to know first aid and not need it than to need it and not know it. Everyone should be able to perform first aid, because most people will eventually find themselves in a situation requiring it, either for another person or for themselves.

A delay of as little as a few minutes when a person's heart stops can mean the difference between life and death. However, most injuries do not require lifesaving efforts. During their lifetime, most people will see only one or two situations involving life-threatening conditions. Although saving lives is important, knowing what to do for the more common and less severe injuries demands greater attention and more first aid training.

▶ What Is First Aid?

First aid is one of those things you need to know but never want to use. <u>First aid</u> is the immediate care given to an injured or suddenly ill person.

First aid does *not* take the place of proper medical treatment. Rather, it furnishes temporary assistance until the victim receives competent medical care, if needed, or until the chance for recovery without medical care is assured. Most injuries and illnesses do not require medical care. **Figure 1-1** shows the leading

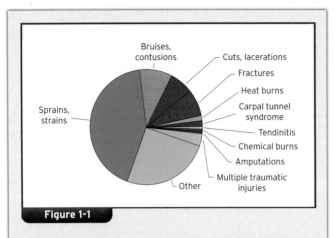

Figure 1-1

Nature of injury or illness of nonfatal occupational injuries and illnesses involving days away from work, 2003.

causes of nonfatal occupational injuries and illnesses in the United States. **Table 1-1** lists the leading causes of death in the United States. **Figure 1-2** compares the number of injuries resulting in death with the number of less severe injuries.

Properly applied, first aid may mean the difference between life and death, between a rapid recovery and long hospitalization, or between temporary disability and permanent injury. First aid involves more than doing things for others; it also includes those things that people can do for themselves.

Recognizing a serious medical emergency and knowing how to get help may mean the difference between life and death. Recognition can be delayed because neither the victim nor bystanders know basic symptoms (eg, a heart-attack victim may wait hours after the onset of symptoms before seeking help). Moreover, most people do not know first aid; even if they do, they may panic in an emergency.

Table 1-1 Leading Causes of Death

Rank	<1	1-4	5-9	10-14	15-24	25-34	35-44	45-54	55-64	65+	All Ages
1	Congenital Anomalies 5,621	Unintentional Injury 1,717	Unintentional Injury 1,096	Unintentional Injury 1,522	Unintentional Injury 15,272	Unintentional Injury 12,541	Unintentional Injury 16,766	Malignant Neoplasms 49,843	Malignant Neoplasms 95,692	Heart Disease 563,390	Heart Disease 685,089
2	Short Gestation 4,849	Congenital Anomalies 541	Malignant Neoplasms 516	Malignant Neoplasms 560	Homicide 5,368	Suicide 5,065	Malignant Neoplasms 15,509	Heart Disease 37,732	Heart Disease 65,060	Malignant Neoplasms 388,911	Malignant Neoplasms 556,902
3	SIDS 2,162	Malignant Neoplasms 392	Congenital Anomalies 180	Suicide 244	Suicide 3,988	Homicide 4,516	Heart Disease 13,600	Unintentional Injury 15,837	Chronic Low. Respiratory Disease 12,077	Cerebro-vascular 138,134	Cerebro-vascular 157,689
4	Maternal Pregnancy Comp. 1,710	Homicide 376	Homicide 122	Congenital Anomalies 206	Malignant Neoplasms 1,651	Malignant Neoplasms 3,741	Suicide 6,602	Liver Disease 7,466	Diabetes Mellitus 10,731	Chronic Low Respiratory Disease 109,139	Chronic Low Respiratory Disease 126,382
5	Placenta Cord Membranes 1,099	Heart Disease 186	Heart Disease 104	Homicide 202	Heart Disease 1,133	Heart Disease 3,250	HIV 5,340	Suicide 6,481	Cerebro-vascular 9,946	Alzheimer's Disease 62,814	Unintentional Injury 109,277
6	Unintentional Injury 945	Influenza & Pneumonia 163	Influenza & Pneumonia 75	Heart Disease 160	Congenital Anomalies 451	HIV 1,588	Homicide 3,110	Cerebro-vascular 6,127	Unintentional Injury 9,170	Influenza & Pneumonia 57,670	Diabetes Mellitus 74,219
7	Respiratory Distress 831	Septicemia 85	Septicemia 39	Chronic Low Respiratory Disease 81	Influenza & Pneumonia 244	Diabetes Mellitus 657	Liver Disease 3,020	Diabetes Mellitus 5,658	Liver Disease 6,428	Diabetes Mellitus 54,919	Influenza & Pneumonia 65,163
8	Bacterial Sepsis 772	Perinatal Period 79	Benign Neoplasms 38	Influenza & Pneumonia 72	Cerebro-vascular 221	Cerebro-vascular 583	Cerebro-vascular 2,460	HIV 4,442	Suicide 3,843	Nephritis 35,254	Alzheimer's Disease 63,457
9	Neonatal Hemorrhage 649	Chronic Low Respiratory Disease 55	Chronic Low Respiratory Disease 37	Benign Neoplasms 41	Chronic Low Respiratory Disease 191	Congenital Anomalies 426	Diabetes Mellitus 2,049	Chronic Low Respiratory Disease 3,537	Nephritis 3,806	Unintentional Injury 34,355	Nephritis 42,453
10	Circulatory System Disease 591	Benign Neoplasms 51	Cerebro-vascular 29	Cerebro-vascular 40	HIV 178	Influenza & Pneumonia 373	Influenza & Pneumonia 992	Viral Hepatitis 2,259	Septicemia 3,651	Septicemia 26,445	Septicemia 34,069

Source: Produced by Office of Statistics and Programming, National Center for Injury Prevention and Control, US Centers for Disease Control and Prevention. Data source: National Center for Health Statistics (NCHS) Vital Statistics Systems. Available at http://webapp.cdc.gov/sasweb/ncipc/leadcaus10.htm.

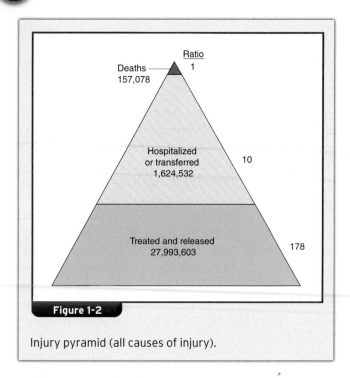

Figure 1-2

Injury pyramid (all causes of injury).

- Of sufficient size to store the needed equipment
- Clearly marked as being a first aid kit by words and/or symbols
- Regularly inspected and updated for completeness and content condition

Workplace First Aid Kit

The following recommended items should be stocked inside a first aid kit for the workplace (Table 1-2). Note that this list does not include over-the-counter ointments, topicals, or internal medicines; consult the workplace's medical director for information regarding these items.

▶ First Aid Supplies

Many injuries and sudden illnesses can be cared for without medical care. For these situations, and for those requiring medical care later, it is a good idea to have useful supplies on hand for emergencies.

The supplies in a first aid kit should be customized to include those items likely to be used on a regular basis. For example, a kit for the home will be different from one for the workplace or for recreational travel.

The supply lists provided in this section include nonprescription (over-the-counter) medications. Some drug products lose their potency over time, especially after they have been opened. Other drugs change in consistency. Buying the large "family size" of a product that you use infrequently may seem like a bargain, but it is poor economy if the product has to be thrown out before the contents are used. Note the expiration date on every medication.

Keep all medicines out of the reach of children. Read and follow all directions for properly using medications. There may be some restrictions on the use of some medications by first aiders without prior written approval (eg, teachers and activity leaders needing parent or guardian permission).

First Aid Kits

First aid kits should be:
- Impact resistant and constructed of a durable material to protect against moisture, dust, and contamination
- Portable and easily carried by a handle

Table 1-2	Sample Workplace First Aid Kit	
Item		**Number to Include**
1. Adhesive strip bandages (1″ × 3″)		20
2. Triangular bandages (muslin, 36″ to 40″, 52″ to 56″)		4
3. Sterile eye pads (2⅛″ × 2⅝″)		2
4. Sterile gauze pads (4″ × 4″)		6
5. Sterile nonstick pads (3″ × 4″)		6
6. Sterile trauma pads (5″ × 9″)		2
7. Sterile trauma pads (8″ × 10″)		1
8. Sterile conforming roller gauze (2″ width)		3 rolls
9. Sterile conforming roller gauze (4½″ width)		3 rolls
10. Waterproof tape (1″ × 5 yards)		1 roll
11. Porous adhesive tape (2″ × 5 yards)		1 roll
12. Elastic roller bandages (4″ and 6″)		1 each
13. Antiseptic skin wipes, individually wrapped		10
14. Medical-grade exam gloves (medium, large, extra large), conforming to FDA requirements		2 pairs per size
15. Mouth-to-barrier device, either a face mask with a one-way valve or a disposable face shield		1
16. Disposable instant-activating cold packs		2
17. Resealable plastic bags (quart size)		2
18. Padded malleable splint (SAM splint, 4″ × 36″)		1
19. Emergency blanket, Mylar		1
20. Paramedic shears (with one serrated edge)		1
21. Splinter tweezers (about 3″ long)		1
22. Biohazard waste bag (3½ gallon capacity)		2
23. First aid and CPR manual and list of local emergency telephone numbers		1

Home First Aid Kit

The American College of Emergency Physicians recommends the following items for a home first aid kit:

1. **Acetaminophen, ibuprofen, and aspirin tablets**—for headaches, pain, fever, and simple sprains or strains of the body. (Note: Aspirin should not be used for relief of flu symptoms or given to children.)
2. **Antihistamine**—relief of allergies and inflammation. Use appropriate dosages and make sure the medicine is age appropriate.
3. **Cough suppressant**—cough relief. Use appropriate dosages and make sure the medicine is age appropriate.
4. **Decongestant tablets**—relief of nasal congestion from colds or allergies. Use appropriate dosages and make sure the medicine is age appropriate.
5. **Antiseptic wipes**—to disinfect wounds or clean hands.
6. **Thermometer**—to take temperature. For babies under age 1, use a rectal thermometer.
7. **Calamine lotion**—relief from itching and irritation from insect bites and stings and poison ivy.
8. **Hydrocortisone ointment**—relief from skin irritation.
9. **Activated charcoal**—treatment for ingestion of certain poisons. (Note: Use only on the advice of a poison control center or the emergency department.)
10. **Elastic wraps**—wrapping of wrist, ankle, knee, and elbow injuries.
11. **Triangular bandage**—wrapping of injuries and making an arm sling.
12. **Scissors with rounded tips**
13. **Adhesive tape and 2″ gauze**—wound dressing.
14. **Disposable, instant-activating ice bags**—for icing injuries and treating high fevers.
15. **Bandages of assorted sizes**—for covering minor cuts and scrapes.
16. **Antibiotic ointment**—for burns, cuts, and scrapes.
17. **Gauze in rolls and in 2″ and 4″ pads**—wound dressing.
18. **Bandage closures, ¼″ and 1″**—taping cut edges together.
19. **Tweezers**—removal of small splinters and ticks.
20. **Safety pins**—fasten splints and bandages.
21. **Medical-grade exam gloves**—protection of hands, reduces risk of infection when treating open wounds.
22. **First aid manual**
23. **List of emergency phone numbers**

Travel First Aid Kit

The American College of Emergency Physicians recommends the following items for a travel first aid kit:

1. **Aspirin, acetaminophen, or ibuprofen**—for headaches, pain, fever, and simple sprains or strains of the body. (Note: Aspirin should not be used for relief of flu symptoms or given to children.)
2. **Antiseptic wipes**—disinfect wounds or clean hands, tweezers, scissors, thermometers, etc.
3. **Calamine lotion**—relief of itching and irritation from insect bites and stings and poison ivy.
4. **Gauze in rolls and 2″ and 4″ pads**—dressing of larger cuts and scrapes.
5. **Antihistamine/decongestant cough medicine**—cough and cold relief.
6. **Antinausea/motion sickness medication**—nausea relief.
7. **Bandages of assorted sizes, including adhesive bandages**—wound dressing.
8. **Adhesive tape and 2″ gauze**—wound dressing.
9. **Elastic wraps**—wrapping of wrist, ankle, knee, and elbow injuries.
10. **Triangular bandage**—wrapping of injuries and making an arm sling.
11. **Scissors with rounded tips**
12. **Medical-grade exam gloves**—reduce the risk of infection.
13. **Disposable, instant-activating ice bags**: icing injuries and treating high fevers.
14. **Antifungal cream (tolnaftate 1% or clotrimazole 1%)**—good for athlete's foot or ringworm.
15. **Antibiotic ointment**—for burns, cuts, and scrapes.
16. **Thermometer with case**
17. **Sunscreen with SPF of 15 or higher**
18. **Insect repellent**—35 to 55% DEET with stabilizer.
19. **Antidiarrhea medications, tablets or liquid**
20. **Antimalaria medications (if indicated)**
21. **Water-purifying pills or liquid (tincture of iodine or halazone tablets) or mechanical filtration devices**
22. **Corticosteroid cream**—for example, hydrocortisone cream; for insect bites.
23. **Tweezers**—removal of small splinters and ticks.
24. **Safety pins**—fasten splints and bandages.

▶ First Aid and the Law

Fear of lawsuits has made some people reluctant to get involved at emergency scenes. Those providing first aid, however, are rarely sued; those who are usually receive a favorable ruling from courts.

Good Samaritan Laws

In most emergencies, you are not legally required to give first aid. To encourage people to assist others who need help, <u>Good Samaritan laws</u> grant immunity against lawsuits. Although laws vary from state to state, Good Samaritan immunity generally applies only when the rescuer is (1) acting during an emergency; (2) acting in good faith, which means he or she has good intentions; (3) acting without compensation; and (4) not guilty of any malicious misconduct or gross negligence toward the victim (deviating from all rational first aid guidelines).

Good Samaritan laws are not a substitute for competent first aid or for keeping within the scope of your training. To find out about your state's Good Samaritan laws, ask for information at your local library or consult an attorney.

Negligence

<u>Negligence</u> means not following accepted standards of care and causing injury to the victim. Negligence involves:

- Having a duty to act
- Breaching that duty (by giving substandard care)
- Causing injury and damages
- Exceeding your level of training

Duty to Act

<u>Duty to act</u> requires an individual to provide first aid. No one is required to render first aid when no legal duty to act exists. Duty to act may occur in the following situations:

- **When your employment requires it.** If your employer designates you as responsible for rendering first aid to meet OSHA (Occupational Safety and Health Administration) requirements and you are called to an injury scene, you have a duty to act. Examples of occupations with job descriptions that may include a duty to act include law enforcement officers, park rangers, athletic trainers, lifeguards, and teachers **Figure 1-3** .
- **When a preexisting responsibility exists.** You may have a preexisting relationship with other persons that demand that you be responsible for them, which means you must give first aid if they need it. Examples include a parent for a child or a driver for a passenger.

When required to give first aid, standards of care must be followed. Standards of care ensure quality care and protection for injured or suddenly ill victims.

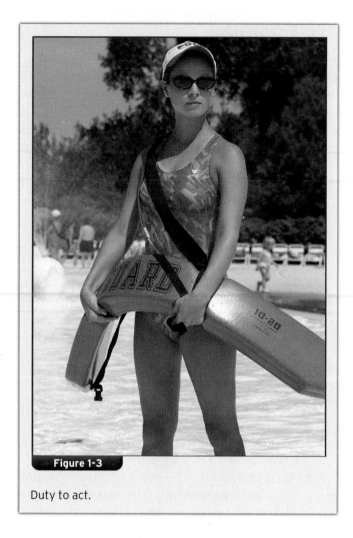

Figure 1-3

Duty to act.

Breach of Duty

A <u>breach of duty</u> occurs when a person providing first aid fails to provide the type of care that would be given by a person having the same or similar training. One's duty can be breached by acts of omission or acts of commission. An <u>act of omission</u> is the failure to do what a reasonably prudent person with the same or similar training would do in the same or similar circumstances. An <u>act of commission</u> is doing something that a reasonably prudent person would *not* do under the same or similar circumstances. Forgetting to put on a dressing is an act of omission; cutting a snakebite site is an act of commission.

Injury and Damages Inflicted

In order to be found negligent, injury or damages must have resulted. In addition to physical damage, injury and damage can include physical pain and suffering, mental anguish, medical expenses, and sometimes loss of earnings and earning capacity.

Consent

Before giving first aid, a first aider must have the victim's <u>consent</u> (permission). Touching another person without that person's permission or consent is unlawful (known as <u>battery</u>) and could be grounds for a lawsuit. Likewise, giving first aid without the victim's consent is unlawful.

Expressed Consent

Consent must be obtained from any alert, mentally competent (able to make a rational decision) person of legal age. Tell the victim your name and that you have first aid training, and explain what you will be doing. Permission from the victim may be <u>expressed consent</u>, and it can be given with words or with a nod of the head.

Implied Consent

<u>Implied consent</u> involves an unresponsive victim in a life-threatening condition. It is assumed or "implied" that an unresponsive victim would consent to lifesaving help. When a child is in a life-threatening situation and the parent or legal guardian is not available for consent, first aid should be given based on implied consent. Do not withhold first aid from a minor just to obtain a parent's or guardian's permission.

Refusing Help

Although it seldom happens, a person might refuse assistance for countless reasons, such as religious grounds, avoidance of possible pain, or the desire to be examined by a physician rather than by a first aider. Whatever the reason for refusing medical care, or even if no reason is given, the alert and mentally competent adult can reject help.

Generally, the wisest approach is to inform the victim of his or her medical condition, what you propose to do, and why the help is necessary. If the victim understands the consequences and still refuses treatment, there is little else you can do. Call EMS, and, while awaiting arrival:

- Try again to persuade the victim to accept care and encourage others at the scene to persuade the victim. A victim could agree to accept care after a short time.
- Make certain you have witnesses. A victim could refuse consent and then deny having done so.
- Consider calling for law enforcement assistance. In most locations, the police can place a person in protective custody and require him or her to go to a hospital.

Abandonment

<u>Abandonment</u> means leaving a victim after starting to give help without ensuring that someone else will continue the care at the same level or higher. Once you have started providing care, you must not leave a victim who still needs first aid until another competent and trained person takes responsibility for the victim.

Confidentiality

First aiders might learn confidential information. It is important that you be extremely cautious about revealing information you learn while caring for someone. The law recognizes that people have the right to privacy. Do not discuss what you know with anyone other than those who have a medical need to know. Some state laws, however, require the reporting of certain incidents, such as rape, abuse, and gunshot wounds.

prep kit

▶ Ready for Review

- Everyone should be able to perform first aid, because most people will eventually find themselves in a situation requiring it for another person or for themselves.
- First aid is the immediate care given to an injured or suddenly ill person. It does not take the place, if needed, of proper medical care.
- The provision of first aid involves a number of legal and ethical issues.
- A person providing first aid must have the victim's consent (permission) before giving first aid.
- Good Samaritan laws offer some protection against a lawsuit when first aid is given voluntarily, the provider expects no compensation, and the care does not deviate from rational guidelines.

▶ Vital Vocabulary

abandonment Failure to continue first aid until relieved by someone with the same or higher level of training.

act of commission Doing something that a reasonably prudent person would not do under the same or similar circumstances.

act of omission Failure to do what a reasonably prudent person with the same or similar training would do in the same or similar circumstances.

battery Touching a person or providing first aid without consent.

breach of duty When a person providing aid fails to provide the type of care that would be given by a person having the same or similar training.

consent An agreement by a patient or victim to accept treatment offered as explained by medical personnel or the person providing first aid.

duty to act An individual's responsibility to provide care to a victim.

expressed consent When a competent patient gives verbal consent or a nod of the head.

first aid Immediate care given to the injured or suddenly ill person.

Good Samaritan laws Laws that encourage individuals to voluntarily help an injured or suddenly ill person by minimizing the liability for errors made while rendering emergency care in good faith.

implied consent An assumed consent given by an unconscious adult when emergency lifesaving treatment is required.

negligence Deviation from the accepted standard of care that results in further injury to the victim.

▶ Assessment in Action

You are driving slowly looking for a house number in an unfamiliar residential area. You are trying to find your friend's new home. While looking for the house, you see an elderly woman lying motionless at the bottom of porch stairs. You see no one else in the neighborhood, and you are alone. You quickly, but safely, stop your vehicle in front of the victim's house. As you approach the victim, you notice that her skin appears bluish.

Directions: Circle *Yes* if you agree with the statement and *No* if you disagree.

Yes No **1.** Do you have to stop to help her?

Yes No **2.** You have implied consent to help this person.

Yes No **3.** If she does not respond to your tapping on her shoulders and shouting, "Are you OK?" you can leave her and assume that someone else who is more competent or is a family member will arrive shortly to help her.

Yes No **4.** You decide to help. Without examining the victim, you quickly straighten her legs, which suddenly causes a bone to protrude through the skin. Would this increase the likelihood of being sued?

Answers: **1.** No; **2.** Yes; **3.** No; **4.** Yes

▶ Check Your Knowledge

Directions: Circle *Yes* if you agree with the statement and *No* if you disagree.

Yes No **1.** Because an ambulance can arrive within minutes in most locations, most people do not need to learn first aid.

Yes No **2.** Correct first aid can mean the difference between life and death.

Yes No **3.** During your lifetime, you are likely to encounter many life-threatening emergencies.

prep
kit

Yes	No	4.	All injured victims need medical care.
Yes	No	5.	Before giving first aid, you must get consent (permission) from an alert, competent adult victim.
Yes	No	6.	If you ask an injured adult if you can help, and she says "No," you can ignore her and proceed to provide care.
Yes	No	7.	People who are designated as first aiders by their employer must give first aid to injured employees while on the job.
Yes	No	8.	First aiders who help injured victims are rarely sued.

Yes	No	9.	Good Samaritan laws provide a degree of protection for first aiders who act in good faith and without compensation.
Yes	No	10.	You are required to provide first aid to any injured or suddenly ill person you encounter.

Answers: **1.** No; **2.** Yes; **3.** No; **4.** No; **5.** Yes; **6.** No; **7.** Yes; **8.** Yes; **9.** Yes; **10.** No

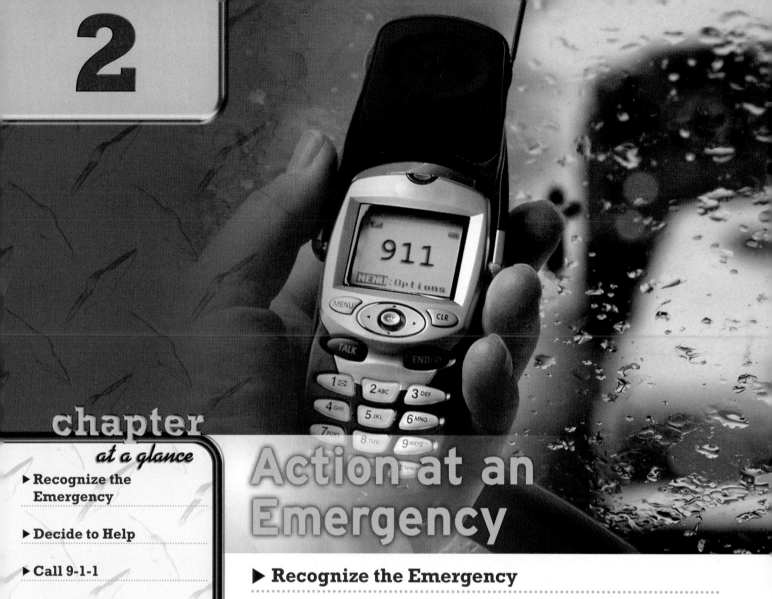

2

Action at an Emergency

▶ Recognize the Emergency

The bystander is a vital link between the <u>emergency medical services (EMS)</u> and the victim. Typically, it is a bystander who first recognizes a situation as an emergency and acts to help the victim. To help in an emergency, the bystander has to notice that something is wrong—usually when a person's appearance or behavior or the surroundings suggest that something unusual has happened.

▶ Decide to Help

At some time, everyone will have to decide whether to help another person. Making a quick decision to get involved at the time of an emergency is unlikely to occur unless the bystander has previously considered the possibility of helping. Thus, the most important time to make the decision to help is before you ever encounter an emergency.

Deciding to help is an attitude about people, about emergencies, and about one's ability to deal with emergencies. It is an attitude that takes time to develop and is affected by a number of factors.

Size Up the Scene

If you are at the scene of an emergency situation, do a quick <u>scene size-up</u>. Such a size up includes looking for three things: (1) hazards that could be dangerous to you, the victim(s), or bystanders; (2) the cause (mechanism) of the injury or nature of the illness; and (3) the number of victims. This survey should only take a few seconds.

First, as you approach an emergency scene, scan the area for immediate dangers to yourself or to the victim. You cannot help another person if you also become a victim. Always ask yourself: Is the scene safe to enter? For details about specific hazards at an emergency scene, refer to Chapter 17.

Second, try to determine the cause of any injury or illness. Be sure to tell EMS personnel about your findings so that they can fully recognize the extent of the problem.

Third, determine how many people are involved. There may be more than one victim, so look around and ask about others involved.

▶ Call 9-1-1

People often make inappropriate decisions regarding calling 9-1-1. They delay calling 9-1-1 until they are absolutely sure that an emergency exists or they elect to bypass EMS personnel and transport the victim to medical care in a private vehicle. Such actions can present significant dangers to victims. Fortunately, most injuries and sudden illnesses that you will render care for will not require the need for advanced medical care—only first aid.

CAUTION

DO NOT call your doctor, the hospital, a friend, relatives, or neighbors for help when a serious condition occurs. Call 9-1-1 in most communities first. Calling anyone else first only wastes time. If the situation is not an emergency, call your doctor. However, if you are in any doubt as to whether the situation is an emergency, call 9-1-1.

When to Seek Medical Care

Knowing when to call for medical care is important. To know when to call, you must be able to differentiate between a minor injury or illness and a life-threatening one. For example, upper abdominal pain can be as minor as indigestion or as severe as a heart attack requiring prompt medical care. Wheezing may be related to a person's asthma, for which the person can use a prescribed inhaler for quick relief, or it can be as serious as a severe allergic reaction from a bee sting.

Not every cut needs stitches, nor does every burn require medical care. It is, however, best to err on the side of caution. **Table 2-1** provides guidance on when to seek medical care.

Table 2-1 When to Seek Medical Care

If the answer to any of the following questions is yes, or if you are unsure, call 9-1-1 or your local emergency number for help.
- Is the victim's condition life threatening?
- Could the condition get worse and become life threatening on the way to the hospital?
- Does the victim need the skills or equipment of emergency medical technicians or paramedics?
- Would distance or traffic conditions cause a delay in getting to the hospital?

The following are specific serious conditions for which 9-1-1 should also be called:
- Fainting
- Chest or abdominal pain or pressure
- Sudden dizziness, weakness, or change in vision
- Difficulty breathing or shortness of breath
- Sudden, severe pain anywhere in the body
- Suicidal or homicidal feelings
- Bleeding that does not stop after 10 to 15 minutes of pressure
- Problems with movement or sensation following an injury
- Hallucinations and clouding of thoughts
- A stiff neck in association with a fever or a headache
- A bulging or abnormally depressed fontanel (soft spot) in infants
- Stupor or dazed behavior accompanying a high fever
- Unequal pupil size, loss of consciousness, blindness, staggering, or repeated vomiting after a head injury
- Spinal injuries
- Severe burns
- Poisoning
- Drug overdose
- Bloody vomiting or diarrhea
- Bleeding that is pulsatile (squirting) or does not stop after 5 minutes of pressure
- Head injury that results in altered consciousness or vomiting
- Severe headache

Immediate care should be obtained if:
- Severe or persistent vomiting
- A gaping wound with edges that do not come together
- Cuts on the hand or face
- Puncture wounds
- The possibility that foreign bodies such as glass or metal have entered a wound
- Most animal bites and all human bites

Source: American College of Emergency Physicians.

How to Call 9-1-1

To receive emergency assistance of every kind in most communities, you simply phone 9-1-1. Check to see if this is true in your community. Emergency telephone numbers usually are listed on the inside front cover of telephone directories. Keep these numbers near or on every telephone. Call "0" (the operator) if you do not know the emergency number.

When you call EMS, the dispatcher will often ask for the following information. Speak slowly and clearly when you provide the following information:

1. Provide your name and the phone number you are calling from. This prevents false calls and allows a dispatch center to call back if disconnected or to request additional information, if needed.
2. Provide the victim's location. Give the address, names of intersecting roads, and other landmarks, if possible. Also, tell the specific location of the victim (eg, "in the basement").
3. Describe what happened. State the nature of the emergency (eg, "My husband fell off a ladder and is not moving").
4. Identify the number of persons needing help and any special conditions.
5. Describe the victim's condition (eg, "My husband's head is bleeding") and any first aid you have provided (such as pressing on the site of the bleeding).

CAUTION

DO NOT hang up the phone unless the dispatcher instructs you to do so. Enhanced 9-1-1 systems can track a call, but some communities lack this technology or are still using a seven-digit emergency number. Because cell phones cannot be tracked through enhanced 9-1-1, it is important that the number be provided to the dispatcher and that all information is conveyed. Also, the EMS dispatcher may tell you how best to care for the victim. If you send someone else to call, have the person report back to you so you can be sure the call was made.

FYI

Actual Versus Perceived EMS Response Time

Patients' perceptions of ambulance response times are inaccurate. They tend to overestimate response time while underestimating scene time and time to medical care.

Source: Harvey AH, Gerard WC, Rice GF, and Finch H: Actual vs. Perceived EMS Response Time, *Prehospital Emergency Care;* 3(1):11-14.

▶ Provide Care

Often the most critical life-support measures are effective only if started immediately by the nearest available person. That person usually will be a layperson—a bystander.

▶ Disease Transmission

First aiders must understand the risk of communicable diseases that can spread from person to person. Such diseases range from mild to life threatening. The risk of getting a disease from a victim is very low. However, first aiders should know how to protect themselves against diseases carried by the blood and air. Precautionary measures help to protect against infection from viruses and bacteria.

Bloodborne Diseases

Some diseases are caused by microorganisms that are "borne" (carried) in a person's bloodstream (bloodborne diseases). Contact with blood containing such microorganisms may cause infection. Of the many bloodborne pathogens, three pose significant health threats to first aiders: hepatitis B virus (HBV), hepatitis C virus (HCV), and human immunodeficiency virus (HIV). Hepatitis is a viral infection of the liver. Types A, B, and C are seen most often. Each is caused by a different virus.

A vaccine for hepatitis B is available and recommended for all infants and for adults who may have contact with carriers of the disease or with blood. Medical and laboratory workers, police, intravenous drug users, people with multiple sexual partners, and those living with someone who has a lifelong infection are at high risk of contracting hepatitis B (and hepatitis C as well). Vaccination is the best defense against HBV. There is no chance of developing hepatitis B from the vaccine. Federal laws require employers to offer a series of three vaccine injections free to all employees who may be at risk of exposure.

For those who have not been vaccinated, symptoms may appear within two weeks to six months after exposure to HBV. People infected with HBV may be symptom free, but that does not mean they are not contagious. These people may infect others who are exposed to their blood. Symptoms of hepatitis B resemble those of the flu and include fatigue, nausea, loss of appetite, stomach pain, and perhaps a yellowing of the skin.

Hepatitis B starts as an inflammation of the liver and usually lasts one to two months. In a few people, the infection is very serious, and, in some, mild infection continues for life. The virus may stay in the liver, which can lead to severe liver damage (cirrhosis) and liver cancer. Medical treatment that begins immediately after exposure may prevent the infection from developing.

Hepatitis C is caused by a different virus from HBV, but both diseases have a great deal in common. Like hepatitis B, hepatitis C affects the liver and can lead to long-term liver disease and liver cancer. Hepatitis C varies in severity, and there may not be any symptoms at the time of infection. Currently, no vaccine or effective treatment for hepatitis C is available.

A person infected with the human immunodeficiency virus (HIV) can infect others, and persons infected with HIV almost always develop acquired immunodeficiency syndrome (AIDS), which interferes with the body's ability to fight off other diseases. No vaccine is available to prevent HIV infection, which eventually proves fatal. The best defense against AIDS is to avoid becoming infected.

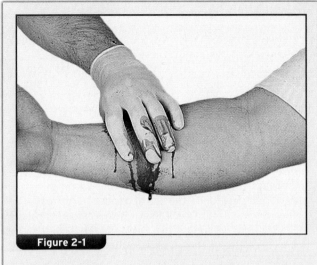

Figure 2-1

Whenever possible, use medical exam gloves as a barrier.

FYI

What Is the Risk of HIV Transmission from Contacting Infected Blood?

In professional football, there are almost four bleeding injuries per game, yet researchers estimate that the risk of HIV transmission in an NFL game is less than one in a million.

Source: Brown LS, et al: Bleeding injuries in professional football: Estimating the risk for HIV transmission. *Ann Intern Med* 122:271-274.

Airborne Diseases

Infective organisms such as bacteria or viruses that are introduced into the air by coughing or sneezing are referred to as airborne diseases. Droplets of mucus that carry those bacteria or viruses can then be inhaled by other individuals. Tuberculosis (TB), a chronic bacterial disease, sometimes settles in the lungs and can be fatal. The rate of TB has increased recently and is receiving much attention. In most cases, a first aider will not know that a victim has TB.

Assume that any person with a cough, especially one who is in a nursing home or a shelter, may have TB. Other symptoms of TB include fatigue, weight loss, chest pain, and coughing up blood. If a surgical mask is available, wear it, or wrap a handkerchief over your nose and mouth.

Protection

Personal protective equipment (PPE) prevents an organism from entering the body. The most common type of protection is medical exam gloves **Figure 2-1** .

The Food and Drug Administration (FDA), the Centers for Disease Control and Prevention (CDC), and the Occupational Safety and Health Administration (OSHA) have stated that both vinyl and latex medical exam gloves provide adequate protection. People who are allergic to latex can wear vinyl or nitrile gloves. All first aid kits should contain several pairs of medical exam gloves.

FYI

Latex Allergies: A Growing Risk

Allergies to latex, or natural rubber, can be disabling, and even life threatening, producing reactions ranging from mild dermatitis to wheezing, urticaria (skin eruptions with intense itching), and anaphylaxis (life-threatening anaphylactic shock). With the emphasis on protection against HIV and other bloodborne pathogens, latex products are becoming very common, increasing the opportunities for and likelihood of exposure to latex. Alternatives to latex examination gloves are products made of nitrile, neoprene, or vinyl. Latex allergy may be a serious barrier to pursuing a career in health care. For those in the health care field who are severely allergic and react even to latex particles in the air, the only option may be to abandon the field of health care.

Source: Kolsun J: Latex allergies: A growing risk. *Emerg Med* 30:66, 71.

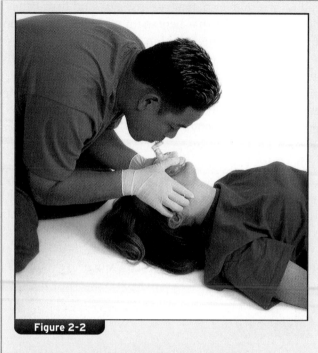

Figure 2-2

Mouth-to-barrier devices are recommended for CPR.

Protective eyewear and a standard surgical mask may be necessary at some emergencies; first aiders ordinarily will not have or need such equipment.

Mouth-to-barrier devices are recommended for rescue breathing and cardiopulmonary resuscitation (CPR) **Figure 2-2**. No cases of disease transmission to a rescuer as a result of performing unprotected CPR on an infected victim have been documented. Nevertheless, a mouth-to-barrier device should be used whenever possible.

Universal Precautions and Body Substance Isolation Techniques

Individuals infected with HBV or HIV may not show symptoms and may not even know they are infectious. For that reason, all human blood and body fluids should be considered infectious, and precautions should be taken to avoid contact. The <u>body substance isolation (BSI)</u> technique assumes that any body fluid is a possible risk. EMS personnel routinely follow BSI procedures, even if blood or body fluids are not visible.

OSHA requires any company with employees who are expected to give first aid in an emergency to follow <u>universal precautions</u>, which assume that all blood and certain body fluids pose a risk for transmission of HBV and HIV. OSHA defines an employee who assists another with a nosebleed or a cut as a "Good Samaritan." Such acts, however, are not considered occupational exposure unless the employee who provided the assistance is a member of a first aid team or is designated or expected to render first aid as part of his or her job. In essence, OSHA's requirement excludes unassigned employees who perform unanticipated first aid.

Whenever there is a chance that you could be exposed to bloodborne pathogens, your employer must provide appropriate PPE, which might include eye protection, medical exam gloves, gowns, and masks. The PPE must be accessible, and your employer must provide training to help you choose the right PPE for your work.

Although EMS personnel follow BSI procedures and OSHA requires designated worksite first aiders to follow universal precautions, what should a typical first aider do? It makes sense for first aiders to follow BSI procedures and assume that all blood and body fluids are infectious and follow appropriate protective measures.

When tending to an injury or illness, first aiders can protect themselves and others against bloodborne pathogens by following these steps:

1. Wear appropriate PPE, such as gloves.
2. If you have been trained in the correct procedures, use absorbent barriers to soak up blood or other infectious materials.
3. Clean the spill area with an appropriate disinfecting solution, such as diluted bleach.
4. Discard contaminated materials in an appropriate waste disposal container.

If you have been exposed to blood or body fluids:

1. Use soap and water to wash the parts of your body that have been contaminated.

2. Report the incident to your supervisor, if the exposure happens while at work. Otherwise, contact your personal physician. Early action can prevent the development of hepatitis B and enable those affected to track potential HIV infection.

The best protection against disease is to use the safeguards described. By following these guidelines, first aiders can decrease their chances of contracting bloodborne illnesses.

▶ Rescuer Reactions

After providing care for serious conditions, first aiders may feel an emotional "letdown," which is frequently overlooked. Discussing your feelings, fears, and reactions following the event can help prevent later emotional problems. You can talk to a trusted friend, a mental health professional, or a member of the clergy. Bringing out your feelings quickly may help to relieve personal anxieties and stress.

prep kit

▶ Ready for Review

- Bystanders are a vital link between EMS and the victim.
- Victims benefit if bystanders can quickly do the following:
  - Recognize the emergency
  - Decide to help
  - Call 9-1-1, if EMS is needed
  - Check the victim
  - Give needed first aid
- First aiders should take BSI precautions to protect against communicable diseases.
- Some incidents can adversely affect the emotional well-being of a first aider.

▶ Vital Vocabulary

<u>airborne diseases</u> Infections transmitted through the air, such as tuberculosis.

<u>bloodborne diseases</u> Infections transmitted through the blood, such as HIV or hepatitis B.

<u>body substance isolation (BSI)</u> Procedures that treat all bodily fluids as potentially infectious.

<u>communicable disease</u> Diseases that can be spread from person to person or from animal to person.

<u>emergency medical services (EMS)</u> A system that represents the combined efforts of several professionals and agencies to provide emergency medical care.

<u>hepatitis</u> A viral infection of the liver.

<u>hepatitis B virus (HBV)</u> A viral infection of the liver for which a vaccine is available.

<u>hepatitis C virus (HCV)</u> A viral infection of the liver for which no vaccine is available.

<u>human immunodeficiency virus (HIV)</u> The virus that can cause acquired immunodeficiency syndrome (AIDS).

<u>personal protective equipment (PPE)</u> Equipment, such as medical exam gloves, used to block the entry of an organism into the body.

<u>scene size-up</u> Steps taken when approaching an emergency scene. Steps include checking for hazards, noting the cause of the injury or illness, and determining the number of victims.

<u>tuberculosis (TB)</u> A bacterial disease, usually affecting the lungs.

<u>universal precautions</u> Protective measures that have traditionally been developed by the Centers for Disease Control and Prevention (CDC) for use in dealing with objects, blood, body fluids, or other potential exposure risks of communicable disease.

▶ Assessment in Action

You are rushing to an important appointment and are running five minutes late. It's beginning to rain and the rush hour is about to begin. Suddenly, you see a motorcyclist skid off the highway and into a ditch. You have a cellular telephone in your car.

Directions: Circle *Yes* if you agree with the statement and *No* if you disagree.

Yes No 1. As you approach the victim, you should not be concerned about any other possible victims.

Yes No 2. This crash scene could be dangerous.

Yes No 3. In most communities, 9-1-1 can be used to contact the EMS.

Yes No 4. Expect to give your name when you call 9-1-1.

Answers: 1. No; 2. Yes; 3. Yes; 4. Yes

▶ Check Your Knowledge

Directions: Circle *Yes* if you agree with the statement and *No* if you disagree.

Yes No 1. A scene survey should be done before giving first aid to an injured victim.

Yes No 2. For a severely injured victim, call the victim's doctor before calling for an ambulance.

Yes No 3. Dial "0" (for the telephone operator) if you do not know the emergency telephone number.

Yes No 4. First aiders should assume that blood and all body fluids are infectious.

Yes No 5. If you are exposed to blood while on the job, report it to your supervisor, and if off the job, to your personal physician.

Yes No 6. First aid kits should contain medical exam gloves.

Yes No 7. Wash your hands with soap and water after giving first aid.

Yes No 8. Vaccinations are available for both HBV and HCV.

Yes No 9. Medical exam gloves can be made of almost any material as long as they fit the hand well.

Yes No 10. Tuberculosis is a bloodborne disease.

Answers: 1. Yes; 2. No; 3. Yes; 4. Yes; 5. Yes; 6. Yes; 7. Yes; 8. No; 9. No; 10. No

Finding Out What's Wrong

▶ Checking the Victim

Checking the victim is an important first aid skill. It requires an understanding of each assessment step as well as decision-making skills. Every time you encounter a victim, first check the scene. The scene size-up determines the safety of the scene, the victim's cause of injury or nature of illness, and the number of victims. Without a scene size-up, a potentially dangerous situation could result in further injury to the victim or to you and others.

The scene size-up is followed by the initial victim check. During the initial victim check, the first aider identifies and corrects immediate life-threatening conditions—breathing difficulties or severe bleeding. Victims with immediate life-threatening conditions can die within minutes if their problems are not quickly recognized and corrected. Determining the type of injury or illness is also part of the initial check.

A physical examination and SAMPLE history follow the initial check. These steps can reveal information that will help identify the injury or illness, its severity, and appropriate first aid. Detailed information is gained about the victim's injury (eg, painful ankle, bleeding nose) or chief complaint (eg, chest pain, itchy skin).

If two or more people are injured, attend to the quiet one first. A quiet victim might not be breathing or have a heartbeat. A victim who is talking, crying, or otherwise alert is obviously breathing.

FYI

Verbal First Aid: What to Say to a Victim

Use these guidelines for gaining rapport and calming injured and ill victims:

1. Avoid negative statements that may add to a victim's distress and anxiety.
2. Your first words to a victim are very important.
3. Do not ask unnecessary questions unless it aids treatment or satisfies the victim's need to talk.
4. Tears and/or laughter can be normal—let the victim know this if such responses seem to make him or her feel embarrassed.
5. Stress the positive (eg, instead of "you will not have any pain," say "the worst is over").
6. Do not deny the obvious (eg, instead of saying that "there is nothing wrong," say that "you've had quite a fall and probably don't feel too good, but we're going to look after you; you'll soon be feeling better").
7. Use the victim's name while providing first aid.

▶ Initial Check

The goal of the initial check is to determine whether there are life-threatening problems that require quick care. This check involves evaluating the victim's breathing, and looking for severe bleeding. By the end of the initial check, the victim's problem will most likely be identified as being an injury or an illness. The following step-by-step initial assessment should not be changed. It takes less than a minute to complete, unless first aid is required at any point **Skill Drill 3-1** :

1. Determine if the victim is responsive: Call the victim in a tone of voice that is loud enough for the victim to hear. If the victim does not respond to the sound of your voice, gently tap the victim's shoulder (**Step ①**).
2. Ensure that the victim's airway is open: In the case of an unresponsive victim, open the airway by using the head tilt–chin lift technique (**Step ②**).
3. Determine if the victim is breathing: Look, listen, and feel for signs of breathing (**Step ③**).
4. Check for any obvious severe bleeding (**Step ④**).

Check Responsiveness

If the victim is alert and talking, then breathing and a heartbeat are present. Ask the victim his or her name

and what happened. If the victim responds, then the victim is alert. If the victim lies motionless, tap his or her shoulder and ask, "Are you okay?" If there is no response, the victim is unresponsive and someone should call 9-1-1.

Open Airway

The airway must be open for breathing. If the victim is speaking or crying, the airway is open. If a responsive victim cannot talk, cry, or cough forcefully, the airway is probably blocked and must be cleared. In this case, abdominal thrusts (Heimlich maneuver) can be given to clear an obstructed airway in a responsive adult victim. This and other techniques for airway and breathing care are described in detail in Chapter 4.

In an unresponsive victim lying face up, the most common airway obstruction is the tongue. Snoring is evidence of this. First aiders use the head tilt–chin lift method to open the airway for all victims even if a spinal injury is suspected. Refer to Chapter 4 for details. Once the victim's airway is clear of blockage, the initial check can continue.

Check Breathing

This step primarily focuses on whether the victim is breathing or having obvious breathing difficulties. Breathing difficulties or unusual breathing sounds include wheezing, crowing, gurgling, or snoring **Table 3-1** .

Table 3-1 Abnormal Breathing Sounds

Abnormal Sound	Possible Causes
Snoring	Airway partially blocked (usually by tongue)
Gurgling (breaths passing through liquid)	Fluids in throat
Crowing (birdlike sound)	Airway partially blocked
Wheezing	Spasm or partial obstruction in bronchi (asthma, emphysema)
Occasional, gasping breaths (known as agonal respirations)	Temporary breathing after the heart has stopped

skill drill

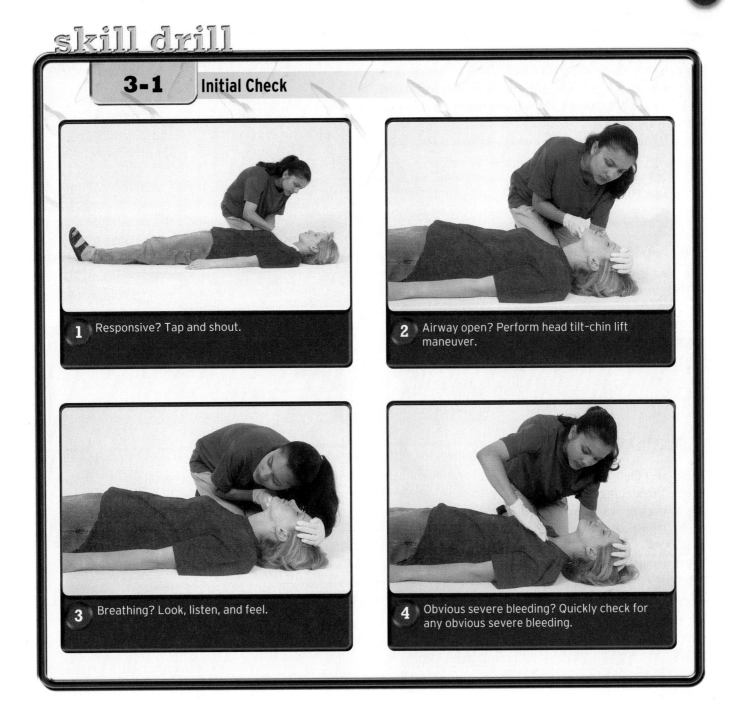

3-1   **Initial Check**

1 Responsive? Tap and shout.

2 Airway open? Perform head tilt-chin lift maneuver.

3 Breathing? Look, listen, and feel.

4 Obvious severe bleeding? Quickly check for any obvious severe bleeding.

Check for breathing in an unresponsive victim after opening the airway. Watch for the victim's chest to rise and fall as you place your ear next to the victim's mouth. "Look, listen, and feel" for about 10 seconds to check for breathing. If the victim is not breathing, keep the airway open and breathe two breaths (each breath lasting for 1 second) into the victim. Refer to Chapter 4 for details. Whenever possible, use a mouth-to-barrier device (mask or face shield).

Check for Severe Bleeding

Check for severe bleeding by quickly looking over the victim's entire body for blood (blood-soaked clothing or blood pooling on the floor or the ground). Controlling bleeding requires the application of direct pressure or a pressure bandage. Avoid contact with the victim's blood, if possible, by using medical exam gloves or extra layers of dressings or cloth. Control bleeding with pressure as described in Chapter 6.

▶ Physical Exam and SAMPLE History

The initial check is followed by a physical examination and the SAMPLE history. During this time you will note the victim's signs and symptoms:

- Signs—victim's conditions you can see, feel, hear, or smell
- Symptoms—things the victim feels and is able to describe; known as the "chief complaint"

Physical Exam

With the initial check complete, and no life-threatening injuries present, perform a **physical exam** to gather information about the victim's condition. To help you eval-

uate these areas, look and feel for the following signs of injury: deformities, open injuries, tenderness, and swelling. The mnemonic DOTS is helpful in remembering the signs of a problem:

- D = Deformities occur when bones are broken, causing an abnormal shape **Figure 3-1**.
- O = Open wounds break the skin **Figure 3-2**.
- T = Tenderness is pain or sensitivity when touched **Figure 3-3**.
- S = Swelling is the body's response to injury that makes the area look larger than usual **Figure 3-4**.

The following are some things you should look and feel for during the physical exam **Skill Drill 3-2**:

1. *Head.* Check for DOTS. Compare the pupils—they should be the same size and react to light. Look for leakage of blood or fluid (cerebrospinal fluid)

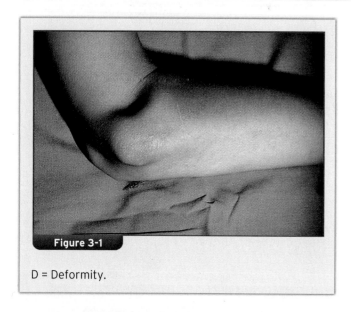

Figure 3-1

D = Deformity.

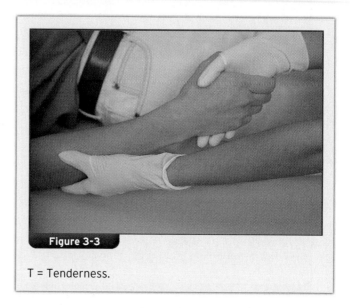

Figure 3-3

T = Tenderness.

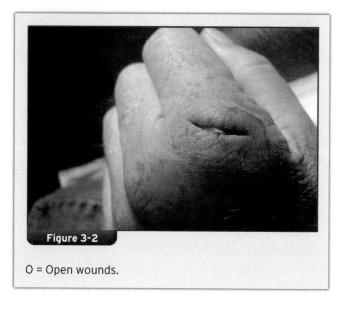

Figure 3-2

O = Open wounds.

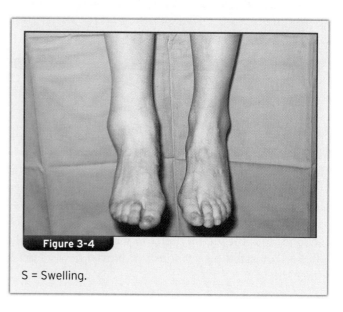

Figure 3-4

S = Swelling.

from the nose or ears. Check the mouth for objects that could block the airway (**Step** ❶).

2. *Neck.* Look and feel for DOTS. Look for a medical identification necklace (**Step** ❷).

3. *Chest.* Look and feel the entire chest for DOTS. Gently squeeze or compress the sides inward together for rib pain (**Step** ❸).

4. *Abdomen.* Look and feel for DOTS. Gently press all four abdominal quadrants for rigidity and tenderness, using the pads of your fingers. If the victim complains of pain in a particular area, ask the victim to point to it; press that area last (**Step** ❹).

5. *Pelvis.* Look and feel for DOTS. Gently squeeze the hips inward together and gently press the hips downward (**Steps** ❺a and ❺b).

6. *Extremities.* Look and feel the entire length and girth of each extremity (arms and legs) for DOTS (**Step** ❻). Check the circulation, sensation, and movement (use the mnemonic CSM as a way of remembering) of each extremity. Check for circulation in the arms by feeling for the radial pulse on the victim's thumb side of the wrist. Check the circulation of the legs by feeling for the posterior tibial pulse between the inside of the ankle bone and the Achilles tendon. In a responsive victim, check for sensation by asking the victim whether he or she can feel you pinching his or her fingers and toes. To check for movement, ask the victim to wiggle his or her fingers and toes. To check for a spinal injury, ask the victim to squeeze your hand with his or her hands, and to push his or her feet against your hand in addition to checking for sensation and movement. Compare the responses of one extremity against the responses of the other for any differences. Lack of sensation or movement can indicate an injured extremity or spinal injury. If you suspect a spinal injury, do not move the victim's head or neck. Stabilize the victim against any movement, and be sure to tell him or her not to move.

CAUTION

DO NOT aggravate injuries or contaminate wounds.
DO NOT move a victim with a possible spinal injury.

Medical Identification Tags

Look for medical identification tags, which may be beneficial in identifying allergies, medications, or medical history. A medical-alert tag, worn as a necklace or as a bracelet, contains the wearer's medical problem(s) and a 24-hour telephone number that offers, in case of an emergency, access to the victim's medical history plus names of doctors and close relatives. Necklaces and bracelets are durable, instantly recognizable, and less likely than cards to be separated from the victim in an emergency **Figure 3-5**.

SAMPLE History

An alert victim may provide information that indicates what is wrong and communicate the need for first aid. The mnemonic SAMPLE helps you remember what information to gather **Table 3-2**. If the victim is unresponsive, you may be able to obtain the <u>SAMPLE history</u> information from family, friends, or bystanders.

Physical Exam and SAMPLE History for Injured Victims

For an injured victim, start by reconsidering the cause (mechanism) of injury that you identified previously, during the scene size-up. This allows you to determine which procedures to use in checking an injured victim.

Injured Victim with a Significant Cause (Mechanism) of Injury

For an injured victim with a significant cause (mechanism) of injury **Table 3-3**, stabilize the head (if the

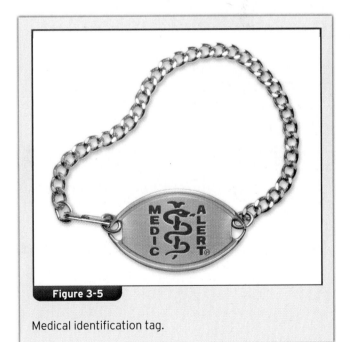

Figure 3-5

Medical identification tag.

skill drill

3-2   **Physical Exam**

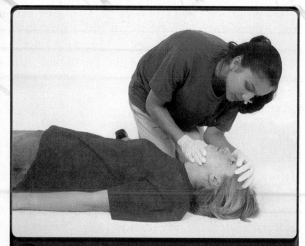

1 *Head:* Check for DOTS. Compare the pupils—they should be the same size and react to light. Check the ears and nose for clear or blood-tinged fluid. Check the mouth for objects that could block the airway such as broken teeth.

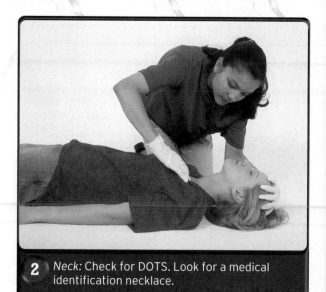

2 *Neck:* Check for DOTS. Look for a medical identification necklace.

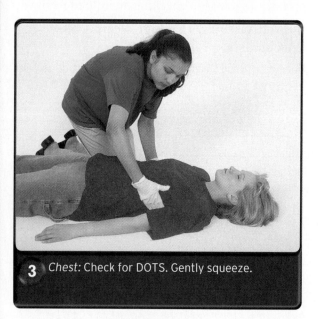

3 *Chest:* Check for DOTS. Gently squeeze.

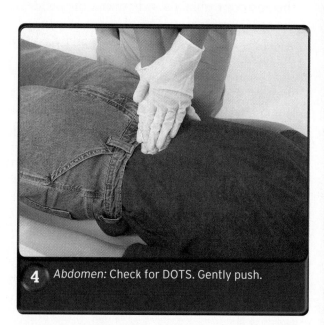

4 *Abdomen:* Check for DOTS. Gently push.

skill drill

3-2 Physical Exam

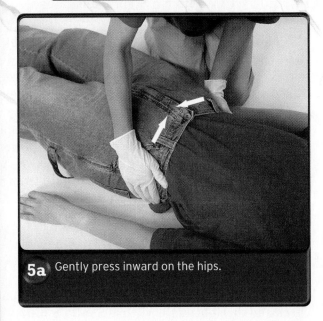

5a Gently press inward on the hips.

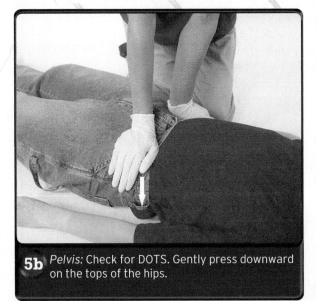

5b *Pelvis:* Check for DOTS. Gently press downward on the tops of the hips.

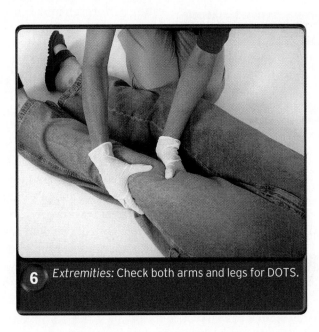

6 *Extremities:* Check both arms and legs for DOTS.

Table 3-2 SAMPLE History

Description	Questions
S = Symptoms	"What's wrong?"
A = Allergies	"Are you allergic to anything?"
M = Medications	"Are you taking any medications? What are they for?"
P = Past medical history	"Have you had this problem problem before? Do you have other medical problems?"
L = Last oral intake	"When did you last eat or drink anything?"
E = Events leading up to the illness or injury	Injury: "How did you get hurt?" Illness: "What were you doing before the illness started?"

Table 3-3   Significant Causes of Injury

- Falls of more than 15 feet for adults, more than 10 feet for children, or more than three times the victim's height
- Vehicle collisions involving ejection, a rollover, high speed, a pedestrian, a motorcycle, or a bicycle
- Unresponsive or altered mental status
- Head trauma with altered mental status (V, P, or U on AVPU scale)
- Penetrations of the head, chest, or abdomen (for example, stab or gunshot wounds)
- Major burn injury
- Death of an occupant in the same vehicle

injury involves the head, neck, chest, or back) to keep it from moving, check breathing, perform a physical examination from head to toe, and, if possible, obtain a SAMPLE history.

Injured Victim With No Significant Cause (Mechanism) of Injury

The physical examination of a victim without a significant cause (mechanism) of injury should focus on the area(s) that the victim complains about. However, make sure that a quick initial check clears any life-threatening conditions. Determine the chief complaint—the problem as the victim describes it. For example, the victim might complain of "twisting" an ankle. Begin the physical examination at the location of the injury using the mnemonic DOTS. Your examination focuses on just the areas that the victim tells you are painful or that you suspect may be injured. After the physical exam, conduct a SAMPLE history.

Physical Exam and SAMPLE History for Ill Victims

With a responsive ill victim, quickly complete an initial check and then obtain the victim's SAMPLE history followed by a physical examination focused on the victim's chief complaint (symptoms). With an unresponsive ill victim, perform an initial check for life-threatening conditions followed by a rapid physical examination, then complete the victim's SAMPLE history, if possible, from bystanders.

▶ What to Do Until EMS Arrives

The initial check, physical examination, and SAMPLE history are done quickly so that injuries and illnesses can be identified and given first aid and, if necessary, transportation can be arranged. After the most serious problems have been cared for, regularly recheck the victim.

Recheck an alert victim who has a serious injury or illness at least every 15 minutes. Recheck an unresponsive victim or one who has difficulties with airway, breathing, or major blood loss or has a significant cause (mechanism) of injury every 5 minutes. Report your findings to EMS personnel when they arrive.

Victim Assessment

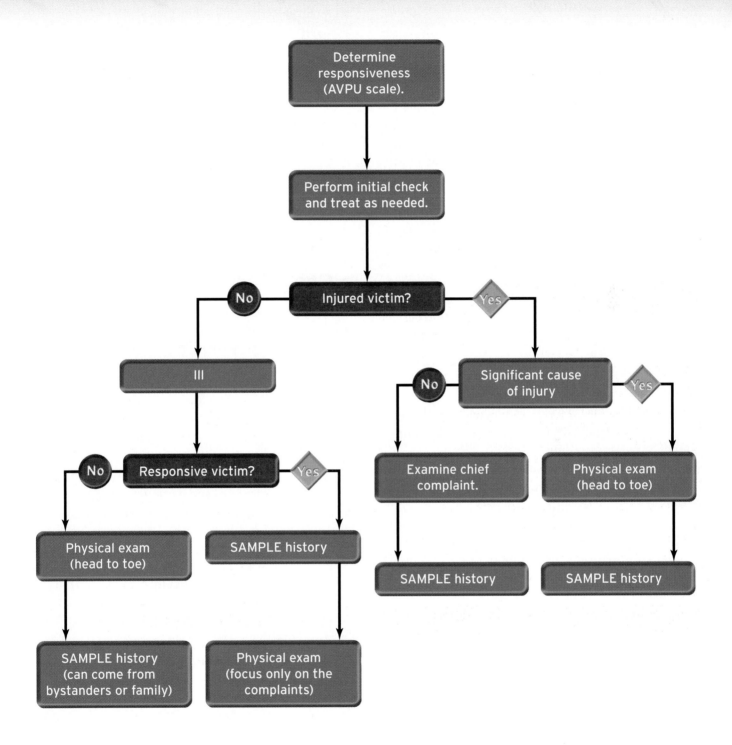

prep kit

▶ Ready for Review

- Determining what is wrong with a victim is essential in providing appropriate first aid.
- Every time you encounter a victim, first check out the scene.
- The initial check determines whether life-threatening problems are present that require quick help.
- The physical exam includes looking and feeling for injuries.
- The mnemonic DOTS helps in recalling what to look and feel for during a physical exam.
- The SAMPLE history gathers information that may indicate what is wrong with a victim and information to be passed along to medical personnel.
- People may have a medical identification tag that can provide information about allergies, medications, or medical history.

▶ Vital Vocabulary

<u>DOTS</u> A mnemonic for assessment in which each area of the body is evaluated for deformities, open wounds, tenderness, and swelling.

<u>initial check</u> A step of the victim assessment in which a first aider checks for life-threatening injuries and gives care for any found.

<u>physical exam</u> Part of the victim assessment process in which a detailed, area-by-area exam is performed on victims whose problems cannot be readily identified or when more specific information is needed about a problem.

<u>SAMPLE history</u> A brief history of a victim's condition to determine symptoms, allergies, medications, pertinent past history, last oral intake, and event leading to the illness/injury.

<u>sign</u> Evidence of an injury or disease that can be seen, heard, or felt.

<u>symptom</u> What a victim tells a first aider about what he feels.

▶ Assessment in Action

The light in the upstairs has gone out, and your roommate doesn't want to wait for the landlord to change the light bulb. He gets a ladder out of the basement and attempts to change the light bulb himself. Unfortunately, he slips and falls off of the ladder while climbing down. You hear a loud thud and run out into the hallway to find your roommate lying on the floor motionless. You notice his medical identification bracelet.

Directions: Circle *Yes* if you agree with the statement and *No* if you disagree.

Yes   No   1. After confirming that the scene is safe, you next check the medical identification bracelet as a clue for finding out what's wrong.

Yes   No   2. If he was unresponsive, you would first look at and then feel his legs for a broken bone.

Yes   No   3. If he was responsive, you would next gather his health history.

Yes   No   4. The physical exam should be started at the victim's head.

Answers: 1. No; 2. No; 3. No; 4. Yes

▶ Check Your Knowledge

Directions: Circle *Yes* if you agree with the statement and *No* if you disagree.

Yes   No   1. The purpose of an initial check is to determine if there are any life-threatening conditions.

Yes   No   2. Victims who are crying or screaming should be treated before quiet ones.

Yes   No   3. Most injured victims require a complete assessment.

Yes   No   4. In a physical exam, you usually begin at the head and work down the body.

Yes   No   5. Tapping a victim's shoulder helps in determining the victim's responsiveness.

Yes   No   6. The mnemonic DOTS helps in remembering what to collect about the victim's history that may be useful.

Yes   No   7. For all injured and suddenly ill persons, look for medical-alert identification.

Yes   No   8. The mnemonic SAMPLE can remind you how to examine an area for signs of an injury.

Yes   No   9. A gurgling sound heard while checking for breathing may indicate fluid in the throat.

Yes   No   10. If during the initial check you find that the victim is not breathing, give two 1-second breaths.

Answers: 1. Yes; 2. No; 3. No; 4. Yes; 5. Yes; 6. No; 7. Yes; 8. No; 9. Yes; 10. Yes

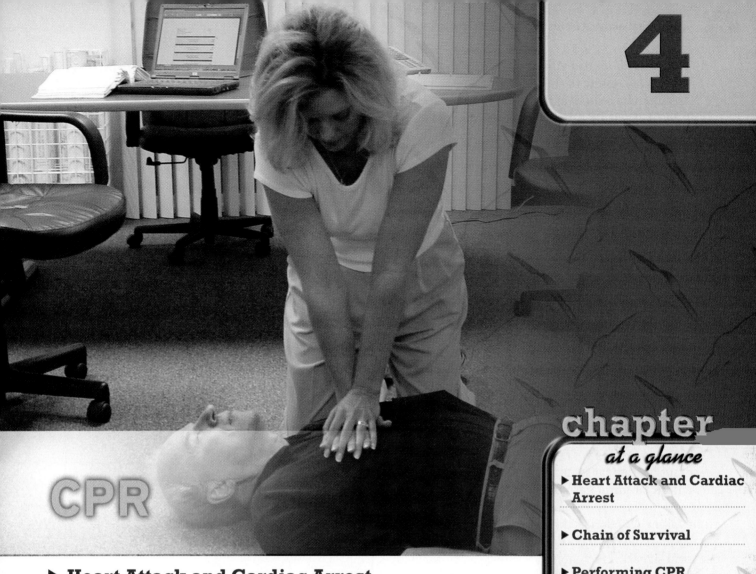

CPR

▶ Heart Attack and Cardiac Arrest

A <u>heart attack</u> occurs when heart muscle tissue dies because its blood supply is severely reduced or stopped. If damage to the heart muscle is too severe, the victim's heart can stop, causing <u>cardiac arrest</u>. This is the most common cause of death in North America. In addition, drowning, suffocation, electrocution, and drug intoxication can cause cardiac arrest. Many deaths can be prevented if the victims receive early <u>cardiopulmonary resuscitation (CPR)</u>, early automated external defibrillation (AED), and early advanced care by trained EMS professionals.

▶ Chain of Survival

Few victims experiencing sudden cardiac arrest outside of a hospital survive unless a rapid sequence of events takes place. The <u>chain of survival</u> is a way of describing the ideal sequence of care that should take place when a cardiac arrest occurs. The four links in the chain of survival are as follows:

1. *Early access.* Recognizing the emergency and immediately calling 9-1-1 to activate emergency medical services (EMS).
2. *Early CPR.* CPR supplies a minimal amount of blood to the heart and brain. It buys time until a defibrillator and EMS personnel are available. It can double or triple the victim's chance of survival.

3. *Early defibrillation.* Administering a shock to the heart can restore the heartbeat in some victims. It can produce survival rates as high as 50 to 75%.
4. *Early advanced care.* Health care providers give advanced cardiac life support to victims of sudden cardiac arrest. This includes providing IV fluids, medications, and advanced airway devices.

If any one of these links in the chain is broken (absent), the chance that the victim will survive is greatly decreased. If all links in the chain are strong, the victim has the best possible chance of survival.

FYI

Defibrillation
Most adults in cardiac arrest need defibrillation. Early defibrillation is the single most important factor in surviving cardiac arrest. Chapter 5 provides information on automated external defibrillators (AEDs).

▶ Performing CPR

One of the leading causes of death in the United States is sudden cardiac arrest, resulting in about 250,000 deaths each year. Most sudden cardiac arrest victims have an electrical malfunction of the heart, which is called *ventricular fibrillation*. In ventricular fibrillation, the heart's electrical signals, which normally induce a coordinated heartbeat, suddenly become chaotic, and the heart's pumping function abruptly ceases. When the heart stops pumping blood, the victim immediately loses responsiveness and is considered clinically dead. A heart in ventricular fibrillation quivers like a bowl of gelatin. When this occurs, the heart is not pumping blood, and only about 4 minutes are available to correct this problem before irreversible brain damage occurs. Without intervention, the victim will become biologically (irreversibly) dead within minutes. When a person's heart stops beating, CPR needs to be performed. CPR consists of breathing oxygen into a victim's lungs and moving blood to the heart and brain by giving <u>chest compressions</u>. Refer to the Skill Drills in this chapter for CPR procedures.

Check for Responsiveness

When the scene is safe, check for responsiveness by tapping the victim's shoulder and asking if he or she is okay. If the victim does not respond, ask a bystander to call 9-1-1. If you are alone with an adult and a phone is nearby, call 9-1-1. If you are alone with an unresponsive child or infant, give CPR for five total cycles (2 minutes), then call 9-1-1.

Open the Airway and Check for Breathing

Before starting CPR, open the victim's airway and check to see if the victim is breathing. Open the airway by tilting the head back and lifting the chin **Figure 4-1**. This moves the tongue away from the back of the throat, allowing air to enter and escape the lungs. The procedure can be done for injured or uninjured victims.

While performing the head tilt–chin lift maneuver, check for breathing by placing your ear next to the victim's mouth and looking at the victim's chest to rise and fall and listen and feel for signs of normal breathing for 5 to 10 seconds **Figure 4-2**.

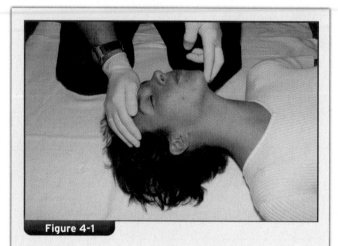

Figure 4-1

The head tilt-chin lift maneuver is a simple method for opening the airway.

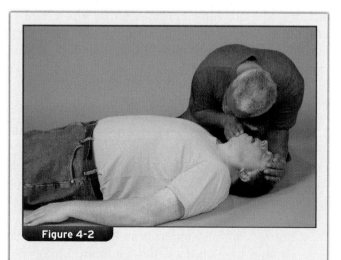

Figure 4-2

Look, listen, and feel for signs of normal breathing.

Rescue Breathing

For the breathing unresponsive victim, place him or her in the <u>recovery position</u>. For the non-breathing victim, rescue breathing must be started immediately. Roll the victim onto his or her back. If a victim is not breathing, perform rescue breathing by using one of the following methods: mouth-to-mouth, mouth-to-nose, mouth-to-stoma, or mouth-to-barrier device.

Mouth-to-Mouth Method

The mouth-to-mouth method of rescue breathing is a simple, quick, and effective method for an emergency situation. Pinch the victim's nose and breathe into the victim's mouth for one second. Take a normal breath for yourself, and then give a another one-second breath. Each breath should make the victim's chest rise.

Mouth-to-Nose Method

Although mouth-to-mouth breathing is successful in the majority of cases, certain complications may necessitate mouth-to-nose rescue breathing; for example, if you cannot open the victim's mouth, their teeth are clenched together, you cannot make a good seal around the victim's mouth, the victim's mouth is severely injured, or the victim's mouth is too large or has no teeth.

The mouth-to-nose technique is performed like mouth-to-mouth breathing, except that you force your exhaled breath through the victim's nose while holding his or her mouth closed with one hand pushing up on the chin. The victim's mouth then must be held open so any nasal obstruction does not impede exhalation of air from the victim's lungs.

Mouth-to-Stoma Method

Cancer and other diseases of the vocal cords often make surgical removal of the larynx necessary. People who have had this surgery breathe through a small permanent opening in the lower part of the neck called a *stoma*, which is surgically made and joined to the trachea.

In mouth-to-stoma rescue breathing, the victim's mouth and nose must be closed during the delivery of breaths because the air can flow upward into the upper airway through the larynx as well as downward into the lungs. You can close the victim's mouth and nose with one hand. Determine breathing by looking at, listening to, and feeling the stoma. Keep the victim's head and neck level.

Mouth-to-Barrier Device

A mouth-to-barrier device is an apparatus that is placed over a victim's face as a safety precaution for the rescuer during rescue breathing. There are two types of mouth-to-barrier devices:

- *Masks.* Resuscitation masks are clear, plastic devices that cover the victim's mouth and nose. They have a one-way valve so exhaled air from the victim does not enter the rescuer's mouth **Figure 4-3** .
- *Face shields.* These clear plastic devices have a mouthpiece through which the rescuer breathes. Some models have a short airway that is inserted into the victim's mouth over the tongue. They are smaller and less expensive than masks, but air can leak around the shield. Also, they cover only the victim's mouth, so the nose must be pinched.

After the barrier device is in place, the rescuer breathes through the device. The technique is performed like mouth-to-mouth breathing. See the Skill Drills in this chapter for the steps for performing rescue breathing.

FYI

Avoiding Stomach Distention

Rescue breaths can cause stomach distention. Minimize this problem by limiting the breaths to the amount needed to make the chest rise. Avoid overinflating the victim's lungs by just taking a normal breath yourself before breathing into the victim. Gastric distention can cause regurgitation of stomach contents and complicate care.

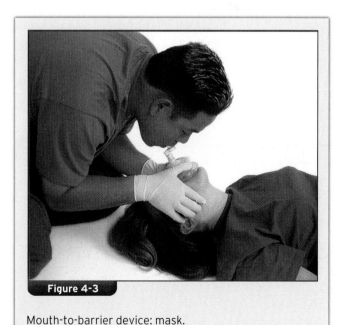

Figure 4-3

Mouth-to-barrier device: mask.

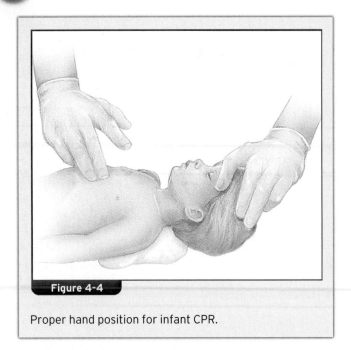

Figure 4-4

Proper hand position for infant CPR.

Chest Compressions

Chest compressions move a small, but critical, amount of blood to the heart and brain. Perform chest compressions with two hands for an adult, one or two hands for a child, and two fingers for an infant. Effective compressions require rescuers to push hard and fast. The chest of an adult should be compressed 1.5 to 2 inches, and the chest of a child or infant should be compressed one-third to one-half the depth of the chest. The chest should be allowed to return to its normal depth after each compression. The desired position for adult and child chest compressions is in the center of the chest between the nipples; for infants, it is just below the nipple line **Figure 4-4**. The victim should be on a hard, flat surface (eg, the floor) and on his or her back.

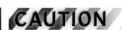 **CAUTION**

First aiders DO NOT:

Check for a pulse or other signs of circulation (eg, movement).

Give rescue breaths without chest compressions.

Use a jaw thrust to open the airway—only health care providers use this maneuver.

Immediately after giving the first two breaths, give 30 compressions at a rate of 100 compressions a minute for all victims (adults, children, and infants). After 30 compressions, give two rescue breaths. Repeat the cycles of 30 compressions and two breaths for five total cycles (2 minutes). Continue the cycles of CPR until an AED becomes available, the victim shows signs of life, EMS takes over, or you are too tired to continue (see Chapter 5 for more information on AEDs).

Over the years, CPR procedures have become easier for people to learn and remember.

To perform adult CPR, follow the steps in **Skill Drill 4-1**:

1. Check responsiveness by tapping the victim and asking, "Are you okay?" If unresponsive, roll the victim onto his or her back.

2. Phone 9-1-1 and retrieve an AED if available, or have another person do this.

3. Open the airway using the head tilt–chin lift method (**Step ❶**).

4. Check for breathing for 5 to 10 seconds by looking for chest rise and fall and listening and feeling for breathing (**Step ❷**). If the victim is breathing, place him or her in the recovery position (see Figure 7-3b). If the victim is not breathing, go to the next step.

5. Give two rescue breaths (1 second each), making the chest rise (**Step ❸**). If the first breath does not cause the chest to rise, retilt the head and try the breath again, and then proceed to the next step. If both breaths cause the chest to rise, go to the next step.

6. Perform CPR (**Step ❹**):
   - Place the heel of one hand on the center of the chest between the nipples. Place the other hand on top of the first hand.
   - Depress the chest 1.5 to 2 inches.
   - Give 30 chest compressions at a rate of about 100 per minute.
   - Open the airway, and give two breaths (1 second each).

7. Give CPR until:
   - An AED arrives and is ready to use
   - Victim begins to move, *or*
   - EMS personnel take over

skill drill

4-1   Adult CPR

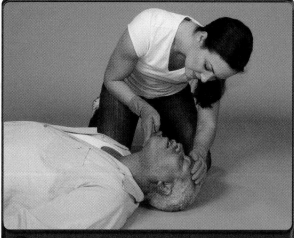

1 Open the airway using the head tilt-chin lift method.

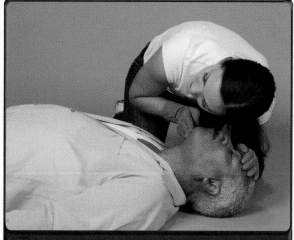

2 Check the victim for breathing for 5 to 10 seconds. If the victim is breathing, place him or her in recovery position. If the victim is not breathing, go to the next step.

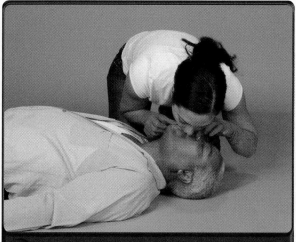

3 Give two rescue breaths (1 second each). If the first breath does not make the chest rise, retilt the head and try the breath again and then proceed to the next step. If both breaths make the chest rise, go to the next step.

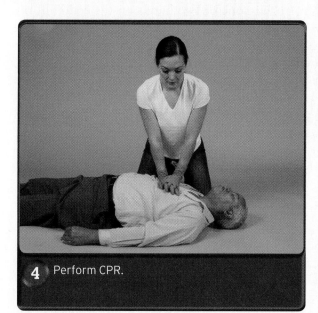

4 Perform CPR.

To perform CPR on a child, follow the steps in **Skill Drill 4-2** :

1. Check responsiveness by tapping the victim and shouting, "Are you okay?" If unresponsive, roll the victim onto his or her back.

2. Have someone call 9-1-1 and retrieve an AED if available. If you are alone, give CPR for 5 cycles, then call 9-1-1.

3. Open the airway using the head tilt–chin lift method (**Step ❶**).

4. Check for breathing for 5 to 10 seconds by looking for chest rise and fall and listening and feeling for breathing (**Step ❷**). If the victim is breathing, place him or her in the recovery position. If the victim is not breathing, go to the next step.

5. Give two rescue breaths (1 second each), making the chest rise (**Step ❸**). If the first breath does not cause the chest to rise, retilt the head and try the breath again, and then proceed to the next step. If both breaths cause the chest to rise, go to the next step.

6. Perform CPR (**Step ❹**):
   - Place one or two hands on the center of the chest between the nipples. If two hands are used, place one hand on top of the other as in adult CPR.
   - Depress chest one-third to one-half the depth of the chest.
   - Give 30 chest compressions at a rate of about 100 per minute.
   - Open the airway and give two breaths (1 second each).

7. Give CPR until:
   - An AED arrives and is ready to use
   - Victim begins to move, *or*
   - EMS personnel take over

To perform CPR on an infant, follow the steps in **Skill Drill 4-3** :

1. Check responsiveness by tapping the victim and shouting, "Are you okay?" If unresponsive, roll the victim onto his or her back.

2. Have someone call 9-1-1.

3. Open the airway by tilting the head back slightly and lifting the chin (**Step ❶**).

4. Check breathing for 5 to 10 seconds by looking for chest rise and fall and listening and feeling for

breathing (**Step ❷**). If the victim is breathing, place him or her in the recovery position. If the victim is not breathing, go on to the next step.

5. Give two rescue breaths (1 second each), making the chest rise (**Step ❸**). If the first breath does not cause the chest to rise, retilt the head and try the breath again, and then proceed to the next step. If both breaths cause the chest to rise, go to the next step.

6. Perform CPR:
   - Place two fingers on the breastbone just below the nipple line (one finger even with the line) (**Step ❹**).
   - Depress chest one-third to one-half the depth of the chest.
   - Give 30 chest compressions at a rate of about 100 per minute.
   - Open the airway and give two breaths (1 second each).

7. Give CPR until:
   - Victim begins to move, or
   - EMS personnel take over

FYI

Compression-Only CPR

Mouth-to-mouth rescue breathing has a long safety record for both victims and rescuers. But fear of infectious diseases makes some reluctant to give mouth-to-mouth rescue breaths to strangers. To avoid the chance that the victim will not receive any care, compression-only CPR can be considered in the following circumstances:

- Rescuer is unwilling or unable to perform mouth-to-mouth rescue breathing.
- Untrained bystander is following dispatcher-assisted CPR instructions.

▶ Airway Obstruction (Choking)

People can choke on all kinds of objects. Foods such as candy, peanuts, and grapes are major offenders because of their shapes and consistencies. Nonfood choking deaths are often caused by balloons, balls and marbles, toys, and coins inhaled by children and infants.

Recognizing Airway Obstruction

A foreign body lodged in the airway may cause mild or severe <u>airway obstruction</u>. In a mild airway obstruction,

skill drill

4-2   **Child CPR**

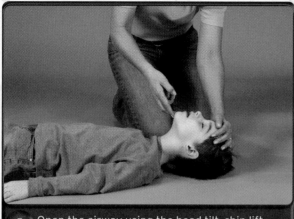

1 Open the airway using the head tilt-chin lift method.

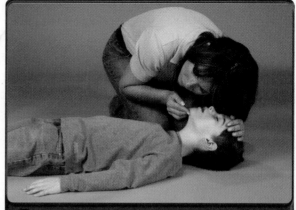

2 Check for breathing for 5 to 10 seconds. If the victim is breathing, place him or her in the recovery position. If the victim is not breathing, go to the next step.

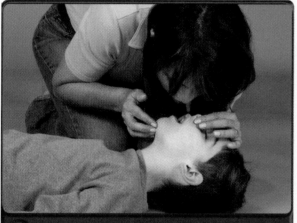

3 Give two rescue breaths (1 second each). If the first breath does not make the chest rise, retilt the head and try the breath again and then proceed to the next step. If both breaths make the chest rise, go to the next step.

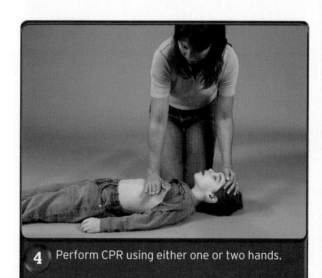

4 Perform CPR using either one or two hands.

skill drill

4-3   Infant CPR

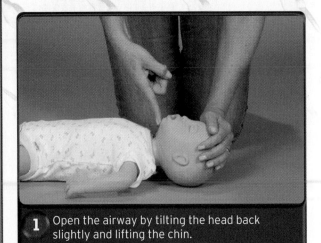

1 Open the airway by tilting the head back slightly and lifting the chin.

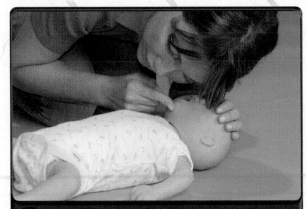

2 Check for breathing for 5 to 10 seconds. If the victim is breathing, place him or her in the recovery position. If the victim is not breathing, go to the next step.

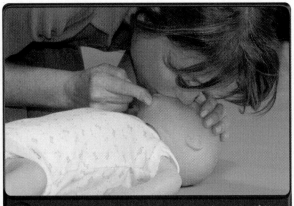

3 Give two rescue breaths (1 second each). If the first breath does not make the chest rise, retilt the head and try the breath again and then proceed to the next step. If both breaths make the chest rise, go to the next step.

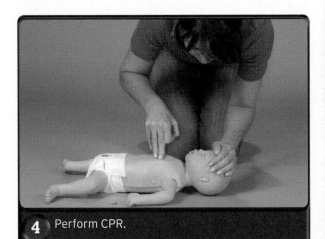

4 Perform CPR.

Adult CPR

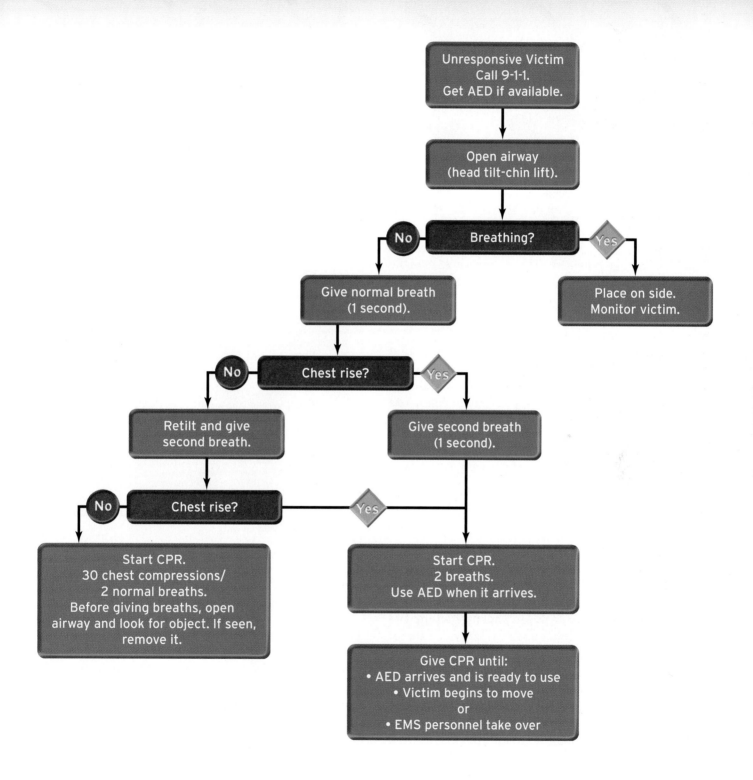

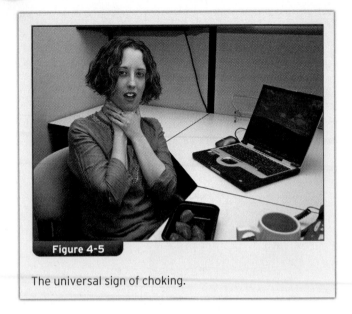

Figure 4-5

The universal sign of choking.

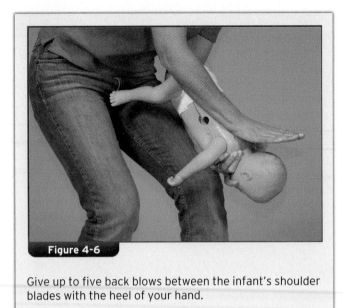

Figure 4-6

Give up to five back blows between the infant's shoulder blades with the heel of your hand.

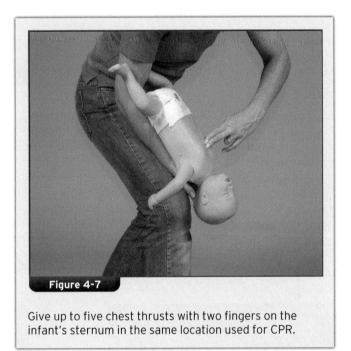

Figure 4-7

Give up to five chest thrusts with two fingers on the infant's sternum in the same location used for CPR.

good air exchange is present. The victim is able to make forceful coughing efforts in an attempt to relieve the obstruction. The victim should be encouraged to cough. Sometimes, however, a mild airway obstruction may progress to a severe airway obstruction.

A choking victim with a severe airway obstruction has a weak and ineffective cough, and breathing becomes more difficult. The skin, the fingernail beds, and the inside of the mouth may appear bluish-gray in color. The victim is unable to speak, breathe, or cough. When asked, "Can you speak?" the victim is unable to respond verbally. Choking victims with a severe airway obstruction may instinctively reach up and clutch their necks to communicate that they are choking **Figure 4-5** . This motion is known as the distress signal for choking. The victim becomes panicked and desperate.

Caring for a Person with an Airway Obstruction

For a responsive adult or child with a severe airway obstruction, ask the victim "Are you choking?" If the victim is unable to respond, but nods yes, provide care for the victim. Move behind the victim and reach around the victim's waist with both arms. Place a fist with the thumb side against the victim's abdomen, just above the navel. Grasp the fist with your other hand and press into the abdomen with quick inward and upward thrusts (Heimlich maneuver). Continue thrusts until the object is removed or the victim becomes unresponsive.

For a responsive infant with a severe airway obstruction, give back blows and chest thrusts instead of abdominal thrusts to relieve the obstruction. Support the infant's head and neck and lay the infant face down on your forearm, then lower your arm to your leg. Give up to five back blows between the infant's shoulder blades with the heel of your hand **Figure 4-6** . While supporting the back of the infant's head, roll the infant face up and give up to five chest thrusts with two fingers on the infant's sternum in the same location used for CPR **Figure 4-7** . Repeat these steps until the object is removed or the infant becomes unresponsive.

If you are caring for an unresponsive, nonbreathing victim of any age and your first breath does not cause the chest to rise, retilt the head and try a second breath. Whether the second breath is successful or not, perform CPR: 30 compressions and two breaths for five cycles (2 minutes). Because the victim may have had a foreign body airway obstruction, look for an object in the victim's mouth and, if seen, remove it before giving the two breaths during the cycles of CPR. To relieve airway obstruction in a responsive adult or child who cannot speak, breathe, or cough, follow the steps in **Skill Drill 4-4** :

1. Check victim for choking by asking, "Are you choking?" (**Step ❶**).

2. If the victim is choking, have someone call 9-1-1.

3. Give abdominal thrusts (Heimlich maneuver). Place a fist with thumb side against the victim's abdomen just above the navel, grasp it with the other hand, and press into victim's abdomen with quick inward and upward thrusts (**Steps ❷ , ❸ , ❹**). Continue thrusts until the object is removed or the victim becomes unresponsive.

4. If the victim becomes unresponsive, check breathing, and give CPR if needed. Each time you open the airway to give a breath, look for an object in the mouth or throat and, if seen, remove it.

To relieve airway obstruction in a responsive infant who cannot cry, breathe, or cough, follow the steps in **Skill Drill 4-5** :

1. Have someone call 9-1-1.

2. Support the infant's head and neck and lay the infant face down on your forearm, then lower your arm to your leg. Give five back blows between the infant's shoulder blades with the heel of your hand (**Step ❶**).

3. While supporting the back of the infant's head, roll the infant face up and give five chest thrusts on the infant's sternum in same location used in CPR (**Step ❷**).

4. Repeat these steps until the object is removed. If the infant becomes unresponsive, begin CPR. Each time you open the airway to give a breath, look for an object in the mouth or throat and, if seen, remove it.

FYI

The Tongue and Airway Obstruction

Airway obstruction in an unresponsive victim lying on his or her back is usually the result of the tongue relaxing in the back of the mouth, restricting air movement. Opening the airway with the head tilt–chin lift method may be all that is needed to correct this problem.

skill drill

4-4   **Airway Obstruction in a Responsive Adult or Child**

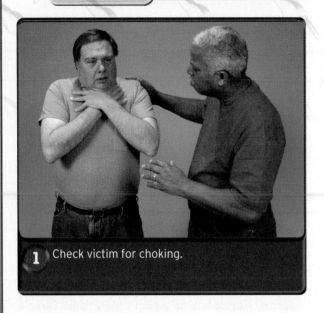

1 Check victim for choking.

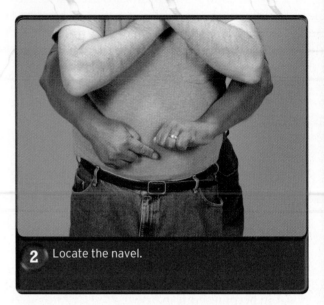

2 Locate the navel.

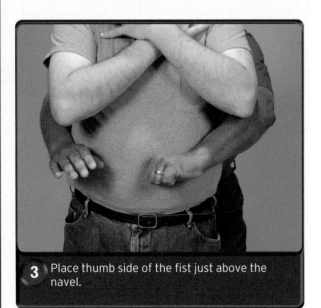

3 Place thumb side of the fist just above the navel.

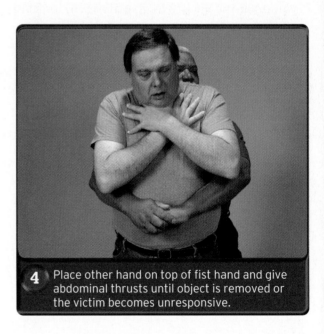

4 Place other hand on top of fist hand and give abdominal thrusts until object is removed or the victim becomes unresponsive.

skill drill

4-5 Airway Obstruction in a Responsive Infant

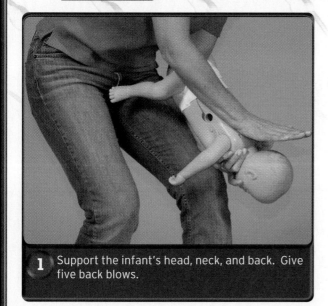

1 Support the infant's head, neck, and back. Give five back blows.

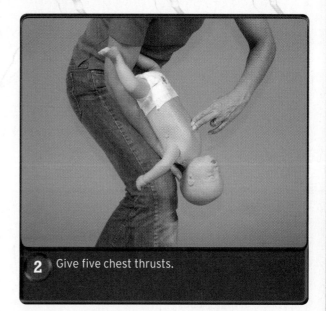

2 Give five chest thrusts.

CPR and Airway Obstruction Review

These eight steps are the same for *all* motionless victims, regardless of age:

- *Check responsiveness:* Tap a shoulder and ask if the victim is okay. If unresponsive, have someone call 9-1-1.
- *Open airway:* Perform the head tilt–chin lift maneuver.
- *Check for breathing:* Look at the chest to see it rise and fall, and listen and feel for breathing (5–10 seconds).
- *If victim is breathing but unresponsive:* place him or her in recovery position.
- *If victim is not breathing:* give two breaths (1 second per breath).
- *If breaths make the chest rise:* begin CPR: cycles of 30 chest compressions and two breaths for five cycles (2 minutes) at a rate of 100 compressions per minute. Recheck breathing after every five cycles.
- *If first breath does not make the chest rise:* retilt victim's head and try a second breath.
- *If the second breath does not make the chest rise (do not give more than two breaths):* assume that the airway is obstructed: Give cycles of 30 chest compressions, look for object in the mouth, remove any visible object, and give two breaths.

Action	Adult (≥8 years)	Child (1 to 8 years)	Infant (<1 year)
1. Breathing methods	Mouth-to-barrier device Mouth-to-mouth Mouth to nose Mouth-to-stoma	Mouth-to-barrier device Mouth-to-mouth Mouth to nose Mouth-to-stoma	Mouth-to-mouth and nose Mouth-to-barrier device Mouth-to-mouth Mouth-to-nose Mouth-to-stoma
2. Chest compressions			
Location	On the breastbone, between nipples	On the breastbone, between nipples	On the breastbone, just below nipple line
Method	Two hands: Heel of one hand on chest; other hand on top	One or two hands (depending on size of victim and rescuer)	Two fingers
Depth	1.5 to 2 inches	One third to one half the depth of the chest	One third to one half the depth of the chest
Rate	100 per minute	100 per minute	100 per minute
Ratio of chest compressions to breaths	30:2	30:2	30:2
3. When to activate EMS when alone	Immediately after determining victim is unresponsive	After performing five cycles (2 minutes) of CPR	After performing five cycles (2 minutes) of CPR
4. Use of AED	Yes; Deliver one shock as soon as possible, followed immediately by 5 cycles of CPR.	Yes; Deliver one shock as soon as possible, followed by 5 cycles of CPR. Use pediatric pads if available.	No
5. Responsive victim and airway obstruction	Abdominal thrusts (Heimlich maneuver)	Abdominal thrusts (Heimlich maneuver)	Alternate five back blows followed by five chest thrusts repeatedly

▶ Ready for Review

- A heart attack occurs when heart muscle tissue dies because the blood supply is severely reduced or stopped.
- The four links in the chain of survival are early access, early CPR, early defibrillation, and early advanced care.
- CPR consists of breathing oxygen into a victim's lungs and moving blood to the brain by giving chest compressions.
- The signs of a severe airway obstruction include the inability to speak or breathe.

▶ Vital Vocabulary

airway obstruction A blockage, often the result of a foreign body, in which air flow to the lungs is reduced or completely blocked.

cardiac arrest Stoppage of the heartbeat.

cardiopulmonary resuscitation (CPR) The act of providing rescue breaths and chest compressions for a victim in cardiac arrest.

chain of survival A four-step concept to help improve survival from cardiac arrest: early access, early CPR, early defibrillation, and early advanced care.

chest compressions Depressing the chest and allowing it to return to its normal position as part of CPR.

heart attack Death of a part of the heart muscle.

recovery position A side-laying position used to help maintain an open airway.

rescue breathing Breathing for a person who is not breathing.

▶ Assessment in Action

You are at a fast-food restaurant and in a hurry to return to work. In a corner booth, a man suddenly gets out of a booth, grabbing his throat and looking distressed. What do you do?

Directions: Circle *Yes* if you agree with the statement and *No* if you disagree.

Yes   No   **1.** Ask the man if he is choking.

Yes   No   **2.** Help the man to lie down.

Yes   No   **3.** If he cannot speak, assume that he is having a heart attack.

Yes   No   **4.** Stand behind the man, wrap your arms around his waist, and give inward and upward abdominal thrusts.

Answers: **1.** Yes; **2.** No; **3.** No; **4.** Yes

▶ Check Your Knowledge

Directions: Circle *Yes* if you agree with the statement and *No* if you disagree.

Yes   No   **1.** If an adult victim is unresponsive, the first aider should call the local emergency telephone number immediately.

Yes   No   **2.** Bending the head back and lifting the chin opens the airway.

Yes   No   **3.** Never touch a victim's face to open the airway.

Yes   No   **4.** When giving chest compressions, push straight down on a victim's chest.

Yes   No   **5.** Perform chest compressions with the victim on a level, firm surface.

Yes   No   **6.** One of the best signs of a severe airway obstruction is that the victim is unable to speak or cough.

Yes   No   **7.** To give abdominal thrusts to a responsive choking victim, place your fist below the victim's navel.

Yes   No   **8.** Before giving a breath to an unresponsive choking victim, check the mouth for an object.

Yes   No   **9.** When giving abdominal thrusts to a responsive choking victim, repeat until the object is removed or the victim becomes unresponsive.

Yes   No   **10.** If the initial first breath did not go into an unresponsive choking victim, retilt the head and try another breath.

Answers: **1.** Yes; **2.** Yes; **3.** No; **4.** Yes; **5.** Yes; **6.** Yes; **7.** No; **8.** Yes; **9.** Yes; **10.** Yes

Automated External Defibrillators

▶ Public Access Defibrillation

Sudden cardiac death remains an unresolved public health crisis. A victim's chances for survival are dramatically improved through early cardiopulmonary resuscitation (CPR) and early defibrillation with the use of an automated external defibrillator (AED). To be effective, defibrillation must be used within the first few minutes following cardiac arrest. The implementation of state public access defibrillation (PAD) laws and the Food and Drug Administration's (FDA) approval of "home use" AEDs have made this important care step available to many rescuers in many places, including the following Figure 5-1 :

- Airports and airplanes
- Stadiums
- Health clubs
- Golf courses
- Schools
- Government buildings
- Offices
- Homes

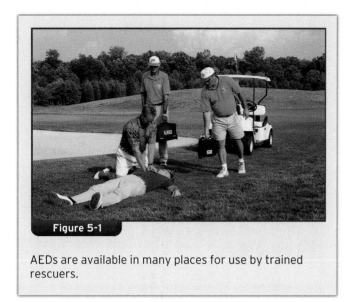

Figure 5-1

AEDs are available in many places for use by trained rescuers.

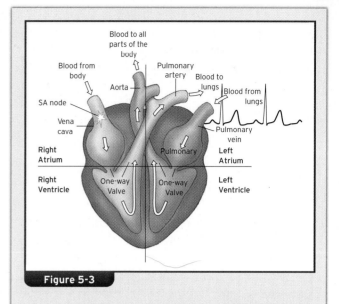

Figure 5-3

The sinoatrial (SA) node is the primary heart pacemaker, which sends electrical impulses to contract the heart's chambers in a coordinated manner.

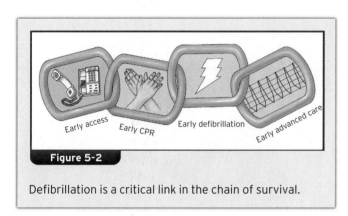

Figure 5-2

Defibrillation is a critical link in the chain of survival.

▶ Chain of Survival

The chain of survival is a concept that recognizes the importance of four critical components in saving the life of a victim of cardiac arrest. Early defibrillation is the third link in this chain **Figure 5-2** :

1. Early access
2. Early CPR
3. Early defibrillation
4. Early advanced care

▶ How the Heart Works

The heart is an organ with four hollow chambers. The two chambers on the right side receive blood from the body and send it to the lungs for oxygen. The two chambers on the left side of the heart receive freshly oxygenated blood from the lungs and send it back out to the body.

The heart has a unique electrical system that controls the rate at which the heart beats and the amount of work the heart performs. The right upper chamber of the heart has a collection of special pacemaker cells. These cells emit electrical impulses about 60 to 100 times a minute that cause the other heart muscle cells to contract in a co-ordinated manner **Figure 5-3** .

Because the heart contracts approximately every second, it needs an abundant supply of oxygen, which it gets through the coronary arteries. These arteries run along the outside of the heart muscle and branch into smaller vessels. These arteries sometimes become diseased (atherosclerosis), resulting in a lack of oxygen to the pacemaker cells, or lack of blood to the heart muscle causing a heart attack.

When Normal Electrical Activity Is Interrupted

Ventricular fibrillation (also known as *V-fib*) is the most common abnormal heart rhythm in cases of sudden cardiac arrest in adults **Figure 5-4** . The organized wave of electrical impulses that cause the heart muscle to contract and relax in a regular fashion is lost when the heart is in ventricular fibrillation. As a result, the lower chambers of the heart quiver and cannot pump blood, so circulation is lost (no pulse). A second, potentially

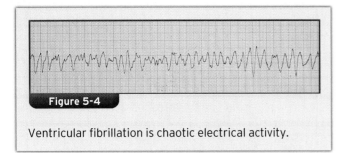

Figure 5-4

Ventricular fibrillation is chaotic electrical activity.

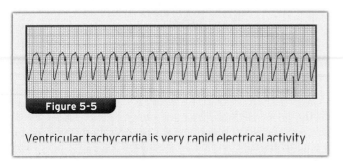

Figure 5-5

Ventricular tachycardia is very rapid electrical activity

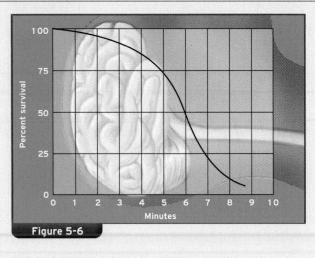

Figure 5-6

A victim's chance of survival decreases with every minute that passes without proper care.

life-threatening, electrical problem is ventricular tachycardia *(V-tach),* in which the heart beats too fast to pump blood effectively **Figure 5-5** .

▶ Care for Cardiac Arrest

When the heart stops beating, the blood stops circulating, cutting off all oxygen and nourishment to the entire body. In this situation, time is a crucial factor. For every minute that the heart isn't beating, the victim's chance of survival decreases by 7 to 10% **Figure 5-6** . CPR is the initial care for cardiac arrest, until a defibrillator is available. Perform cycles of chest compressions and breaths until an AED is ready to be connected to the victim.

▶ About AEDs

An AED is an electronic device that analyzes the heart rhythm and, if necessary, delivers an electrical shock, known as defibrillation, to the heart of a person in cardiac arrest. The purpose of this shock is to correct one of the abnormal electrical disturbances previously discussed and to reestablish a heart rhythm that will result in normal electrical and pumping function.

An AED is attached to the victim by a cable connected to two adhesive pads (electrodes) placed on the victim's chest. The pad and cable system sends the electrical signal from the heart into the device for analysis and delivers the electric shock to the victim when needed **Figure 5-7** .

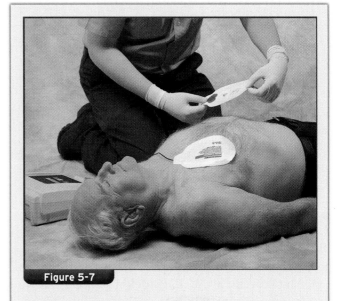

Figure 5-7

Two adhesive pads are placed on the victim's chest and connected by a cable to the AED.

AEDs have built-in rhythm analysis systems that determine whether the victim needs a shock. This system enables first aiders and other rescuers to deliver early defibrillation with only minimal training. AEDs also record the victim's heart rhythm (known as an *electrocardiogram,* or *ECG*), shock data, and other information about the device's performance (eg, the date, time, and number of shocks supplied) **Figure 5-8** .

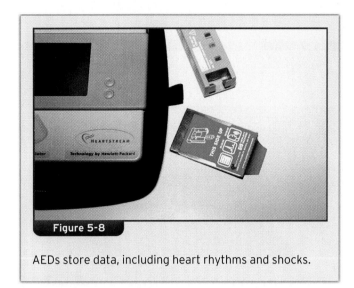

Figure 5-8

AEDs store data, including heart rhythms and shocks.

Common Elements of AEDs

Many different AED models exist. The principles for use are the same for each, but the displays, controls, and options vary slightly. You will need to know how to use your specific AED. All AEDs have the following elements in common:

- Power on/off mechanism
- Cable and pads (electrodes)
- Analysis capability
- Defibrillation capability
- Prompts to guide you
- Battery operation for portability

▶ Using an AED

Once you have determined the need for the AED (victim unresponsive and not breathing), the basic operation of all AED models for anyone over 1 year of age follows this sequence **Skill Drill 5-1**.

1. Perform CPR until an AED is available (**Step ❶**).
2. Once the AED is available, turn the equipment on.
3. Apply the electrode pads to the victim's bare chest and the cable to the AED (**Step ❷**). Use child pads for a child if available.
4. Stand clear and analyze the heart rhythm.
5. Deliver a shock if indicated (**Step ❸**).
6. Perform CPR for five cycles (2 minutes) (**Step ❹**).
7. Check the victim and repeat the analysis, shock, and CPR steps as needed.

Some AEDs power on by pressing an on/off button. Others power on when opening the AED case lid. Once

the power is on, the AED will quickly go through some internal checks and will then begin to provide voice and screen prompts. Expose the victim's chest. The skin must be fairly dry so that the pads will adhere and conduct electricity properly. If necessary, dry the skin with a towel. Because excessive chest hair may also interfere with adhesion and electrical conduction, you may need to quickly shave the area where the pads are to be placed.

Remove the backing from the pads and apply them firmly to the victim's bare chest according to the diagram on the pads. One pad is placed to the right of the breastbone, just below the collarbone and above the right nipple. The second pad is placed on the left side of the chest, left of the nipple and above the lower rib margin.

Make sure the cable is attached to the AED, and stand clear for analysis of the heart's electrical activity. No one should be in contact with the victim at this time, or later if a shock is indicated.

The AED will advise if a shock is needed. Deliver the shock after verifying that no one is in contact with the victim. Begin CPR immediately following the shock for five cycles (2 minutes). Following CPR, recheck to see if the victim is breathing and reanalyze the rhythm. If the shock worked, the victim will begin to regain signs of life. Continue providing care until EMS personnel arrive and take over.

▶ Special Considerations

There are several special situations that you should be aware of when using an AED. These include the following:

- Water
- Children
- Medication patches
- Implanted devices

Water

Because water conducts electricity, it may provide an energy pathway between the AED and the rescuer or bystanders. Remove the victim from free-standing water. Quickly dry the chest before applying the pads. The risk to the rescuers and bystanders is very low if the chest is dry and the pads are secured to the chest.

Children

Cardiac arrest in children is usually caused by an airway or breathing problem, rather than a primary heart problem as in adults. AEDs can deliver energy levels appropriate for children age 1 year or older. If your AED has special pediatric pads and cable, use these for the

skill drill

5-1   Using an AED

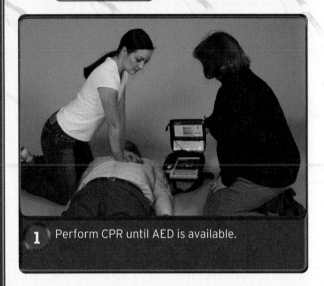

1 Perform CPR until AED is available.

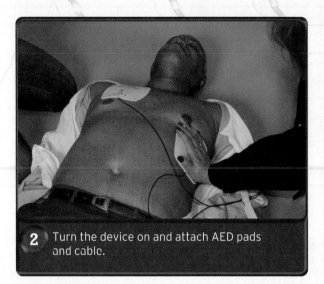

2 Turn the device on and attach AED pads and cable.

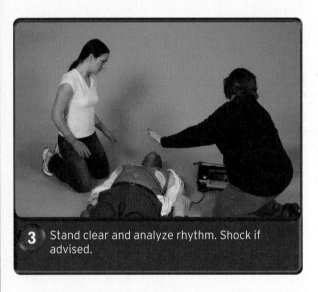

3 Stand clear and analyze rhythm. Shock if advised.

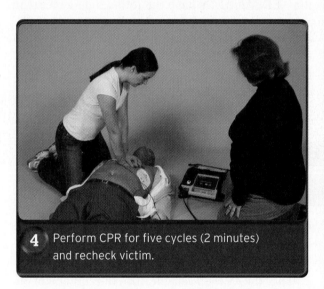

4 Perform CPR for five cycles (2 minutes) and recheck victim.

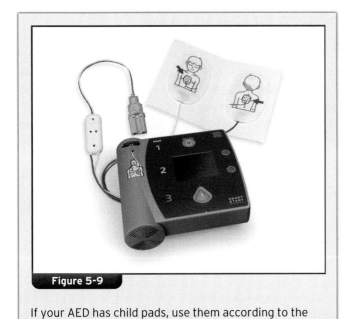

Figure 5-9

If your AED has child pads, use them according to the manufacturer's instructions.

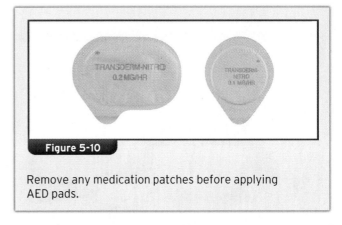

Figure 5-10

Remove any medication patches before applying AED pads.

child **Figure 5-9**. If the pediatric equipment is not available, use an adult AED and pads.

Medication Patches

Some people wear an adhesive patch containing medication (such as nitroglycerin, nicotine, or pain medication) that is absorbed through the skin. Because these patches may block the delivery of energy from the pads to the heart, they need to be removed and the skin wiped dry before attaching the AED pads **Figure 5-10**.

Implanted Devices

Implanted pacemakers and defibrillators are small devices placed underneath the skin of people with certain types of heart disease **Figure 5-11**. These devices can often be seen or felt when the chest is exposed. Avoid placing the pads directly over these devices whenever possible. If an implanted defibrillator is discharging, you may see the victim twitching periodically. Allow the implanted unit to stop before using your AED.

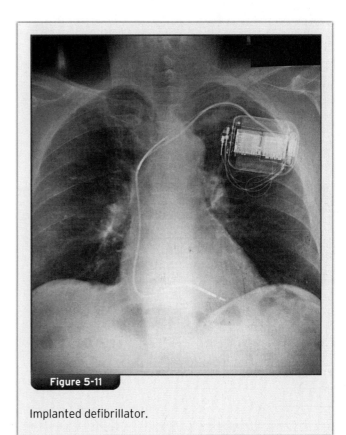

Figure 5-11

Implanted defibrillator.

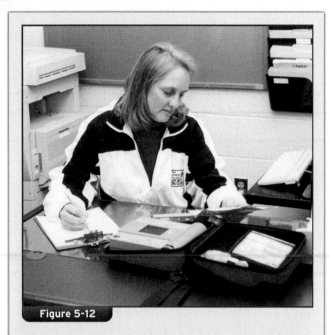

Figure 5-12

Inspect your AED daily to make sure it is working properly and has the necessary supplies.

▶ AED Maintenance

Periodic inspection of your AED can ensure that the device has the necessary supplies and is in proper working condition **Figure 5-12**. AEDs conduct automatic internal checks and provide visual indications that the unit is ready and functioning properly. You do not need to turn the device on daily to check it as part of any inspection. Doing so will only wear down the battery.

AED supplies should include items such as the following:

- Two sets of electrode pads with expiration dates that are not expired
- Extra battery
- Razor
- Hand towel

Other items that should be considered are a breathing device (eg, a mask or shield) and medical exam gloves.

What to Look For	What to Do
Unresponsiveness Not breathing	1. Perform CPR until an AED is available. 2. Turn on the AED. 3. Apply the pads. 4. Analyze the heart rhythm. 5. Administer a shock if needed. 6. Perform CPR for five cycles (2 minutes). 7. Recheck.

AED Skill Checklist

Student's Name _____ Date _____

Skills	Satisfactory	Unsatisfactory
Check for Scene Safety	○	○

Initial check and care:
If two rescuers are involved, one assesses and performs CPR while the other applies the AED.

	Satisfactory	Unsatisfactory
• Establish unresponsiveness.	○	○
• Have someone call 9-1-1 and get AED.	○	○
• Open airway.	○	○
• Check for breathing (5–10 seconds).	○	○
• Give two breaths (1 second each).	○	○
• Give CPR until an AED is available.	○	○

Defibrillation:

	Satisfactory	Unsatisfactory
• Turn AED power on.	○	○
• Ensure skin surface is dry.	○	○
• Apply electrode pads correctly.	○	○
• Ensure electrode cable is plugged in.	○	○
• Stand clear while analyzing.	○	○
• If shock is indicated:	○	○
a. Remain clear.	○	○
b. Deliver shock.	○	○
c. Perform five cycles (2 minutes) of CPR.	○	○
d. Reanalyze.	○	○
• If shock is indicated, repeat steps a through d.	○	○
• If no shock is indicated:	○	○
a. Check victim for breathing.	○	○
b. If victim is not breathing, perform five cycles (2 minutes) of CPR and reanalyze.	○	○

Pass _____   Fail _____

prep kit

▶ Ready for Review

- Sudden cardiac death remains an unresolved public health crisis.
- A victim's chances for survival are dramatically improved through early CPR and early defibrillation.
- The links in the chain of survival are early access, early CPR, early defibrillation, and early advanced care.
- Because the heart contracts approximately every second, it needs an abundant supply of oxygen.
- CPR is the initial care for cardiac arrest until a defibrillator is available.
- An AED is an electronic device that analyzes the heart rhythm and delivers an electrical shock to the heart of a person in cardiac arrest.
- There are several special situations to be aware of when using an AED, including: water, children, medication patches, and implanted devices.
- Periodic inspection of the AED can ensure that the device has the necessary supplies and is in proper working condition.

▶ Vital Vocabulary

automated external defibrillator (AED) Device capable of analyzing the heart rhythm and providing a shock.

defibrillation The electrical shock administered by an AED to reestablish a normal heart rhythm.

▶ Assessment in Action

A 45-year-old professor suddenly collapses during lunch in the cafeteria. You and several other students witness this event. You check the victim and determine that he is not breathing. Your school has recently implemented an AED program, and you and other students have been trained. This person needs your help to save his life.

Directions: Circle *Yes* if you agree with the statement and *No* if you disagree.

Yes No **1.** As soon as you determine that the victim is unresponsive, you should send someone to call 9-1-1 and retrieve the AED.

Yes No **2.** CPR should be performed for at least 2 minutes even if the AED is readily available.

Yes No **3.** The AED pads can be applied over the top of the victim's shirt.

Yes No **4.** If you receive a prompt from the AED that reads "Check Electrodes," the device may be indicating improper placement or poor connection.

Answers: **1.** Yes; **2.** No; **3.** No; **4.** Yes

▶ Check Your Knowledge

Directions: Circle *Yes* if you agree with the statement and *No* if you disagree.

Yes No **1.** The earlier defibrillation occurs, the better the victim's chance of survival.

Yes No **2.** An AED is only to be applied to a victim who is unresponsive and not breathing.

Yes No **3.** CPR is not needed if you are sure an AED will be available in 3 to 4 minutes.

Yes No **4.** AEDs require the operator to know how to interpret heart rhythms.

Yes No **5.** Because all AEDs are different, the basic steps of operation are also different.

Yes No **6.** The AED pads (electrodes) need to be attached to a dry chest.

Yes No **7.** Two electrode pads are placed on the left side of the victim's chest.

Yes No **8.** Batteries and pads have expiration dates you should be aware of.

Yes No **9.** An AED can still be used if an implanted pacemaker is present.

Yes No **10.** You need to turn the AED on daily as part of a routine inspection.

Answers: **1.** Yes; **2.** Yes; **3.** No; **4.** No; **5.** No; **6.** Yes; **7.** No; **8.** Yes; **9.** Yes; **10.** No

Bleeding and Wounds

▶ External Bleeding

External bleeding occurs when blood can be seen coming from an open wound. The term <u>hemorrhage</u> refers to a large amount of bleeding in a short time.

Recognizing External Bleeding

External bleeding can be classified into three types according to its source Figure 6-1 :

- With <u>arterial bleeding</u>, blood spurts (up to several feet) with each heartbeat. It is the most serious type of bleeding because blood is lost at a fast rate, leading to a large blood loss that is difficult to control. Arterial bleeding also is less likely to clot because blood can clot only when it is flowing slowly or not at all. However, unless a very large artery has been cut, it is unlikely that a person will bleed to death before the flow can be controlled. Nevertheless, arterial bleeding is dangerous and must be controlled.
- <u>Venous bleeding</u> flows steadily and is easier to control than arterial bleeding because the blood is under less pressure and does not spurt. Most veins collapse when cut. Bleeding from deep veins, however, can be as massive and as difficult to control as arterial bleeding.
- <u>Capillary bleeding</u> oozes from capillaries. It is the most common type of bleeding. It usually is not serious and is easily controlled. Often, this type of bleeding will clot and stop by itself.

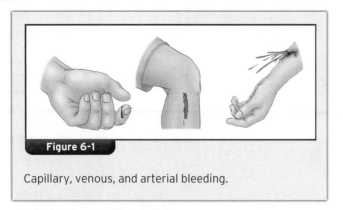

Figure 6-1

Capillary, venous, and arterial bleeding.

There are several types of open wounds **Figure 6-2** :

- *Abrasion.* The top layer of skin is removed, with little or no blood loss. Abrasions tend to be painful, because the nerve endings often are torn along with the skin. Ground-in debris may be present. This type of wound can be serious if it covers a large area or becomes embedded with foreign matter. Other names for an abrasion are *scrape* or *road rash.*
- *Laceration.* The skin is cut with jagged, irregular edges. This type of wound usually is caused by a forceful tearing away of skin tissue.

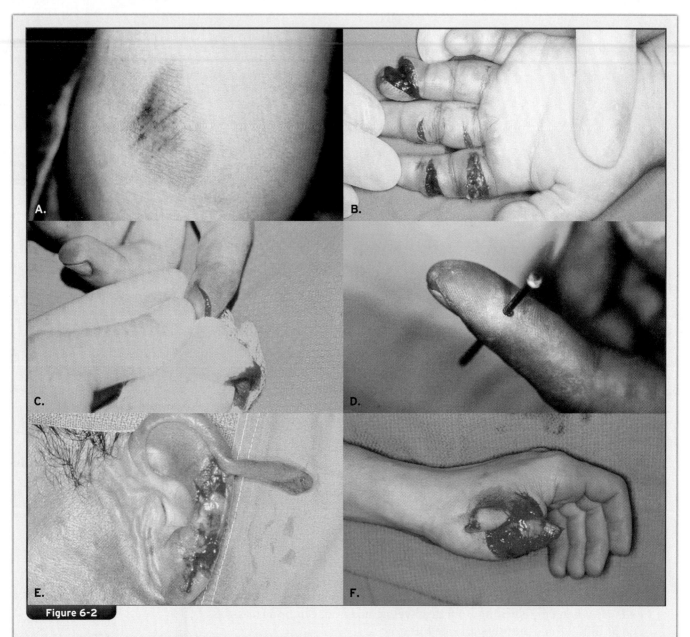

Figure 6-2

Open wounds. **A.** Abrasion. **B.** Laceration. **C.** Incision. **D.** Puncture. **E.** Avulsion. **F.** Amputation.

- *Incisions.* A cut with smooth edges such as a surgical or paper cut. The amount of bleeding depends on the depth, the location, and the size of the wound.
- *Punctures.* These are usually deep, narrow wounds, such as a stab wound from a sharp, pointed object (eg, a nail, knife, or bullet). The penetrating object can damage internal organs. The entrance is usually small, and the risk of infection is high. The object causing the injury may remain impaled in the wound.
- *Avulsion.* A piece of skin torn loose hanging from the body. This type of wound can bleed heavily. The flap of skin should be returned to its normal position. Avulsions most often involve ears, fingers, and hands.
- *Amputation.* This involves the cutting or tearing off of a body part. Amputations most often involve a finger, toe, hand, foot, arm, or leg.

Care for External Bleeding

Regardless of the type of bleeding or the type of wound, the first aid is the same. First, and most important, you must control the bleeding **Skill Drill 6-1** :

1. Protect yourself against disease by wearing medical exam gloves (**Step ❶**). If medical exam gloves are not available, use several layers of gauze pads, plastic wrap, a plastic bag, clean cloths, or waterproof material. You can even have the victim apply pressure on the wound with his or her own hand. After bleeding has stopped and the wound has been cared for, vigorously wash your hands with soap and water.

2. Expose the wound by removing or cutting the clothing to find the source of the blood.

3. Place a dressing such as a sterile gauze pad or a clean cloth (eg, a handkerchief, washcloth, or towel) over the wound and apply direct pressure with your fingers or the palm of your hand (**Step ❷**). Hold steady, firm pressure uninterrupted for at least 5 minutes. This technique stops most bleeding. If blood flow does not stop, apply more pressure, and hold longer. Sometimes, continuous pressure must be held until medical care arrives.

4. If bleeding is from arm or leg, elevate the injured area above heart level as you continue to apply pressure to reduce blood flow (**Step ❸**). Elevating the extremity allows gravity to reduce blood flow and makes it difficult for the body to pump blood to the affected limb.

5. If the bleeding still cannot be controlled in an extremity, keep applying direct pressure over the wound and apply pressure at a pressure point to slow the flow of blood. A pressure point is where an artery near the skin's surface passes close to a bone, against which it can be compressed. The most accessible pressure points on both sides of the body are the brachial point in the upper inside arm and the femoral point in the groin **Figure 6-3** .

6. To free you to attend to other injuries or victims, apply a pressure bandage to hold the dressing on the wound. Wrap a roller gauze bandage tightly over the dressing and above and below the wound site (**Step ❹**).

7. When you cannot apply direct pressure (eg, in the case of a protruding bone, skull fracture, or embedded object), apply pressure around the injured area. One way to do this is by placing the outside edges of your hand around the area and then applying pressure. Another method is to make a doughnut-shaped (ring) pad to control bleeding (see Chapter 9, Head and Spinal Injuries). To make a ring pad, wrap one end of a narrow bandage (roller or cravat) several times around your four fingers to form a loop. Pass the other end of the bandage through the loop and wrap it around until the entire bandage is used and a ring has been made. Place the pad around the injured area and then apply pressure.

8. When bleeding stops, use procedures in the Wound Care section.

CAUTION

DO NOT touch a wound with your bare hands. If you must use your bare hands, do so only as a last resort. After the bleeding has stopped and the wound has been cared for, vigorously wash your hands with soap and water.

DO NOT use direct pressure on an eye injury, a wound with an embedded object, or a skull fracture.

DO NOT remove a blood-soaked dressing. Apply another dressing on top and keep pressing.

skill drill

6-1 Care for External Bleeding

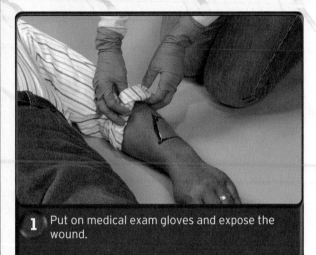

1 Put on medical exam gloves and expose the wound.

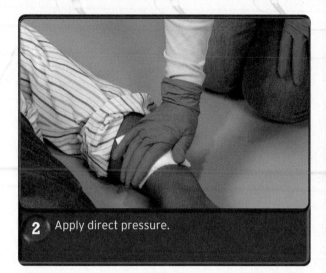

2 Apply direct pressure.

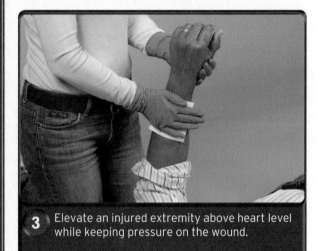

3 Elevate an injured extremity above heart level while keeping pressure on the wound.

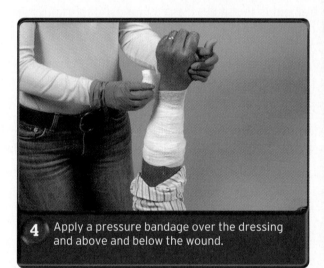

4 Apply a pressure bandage over the dressing and above and below the wound.

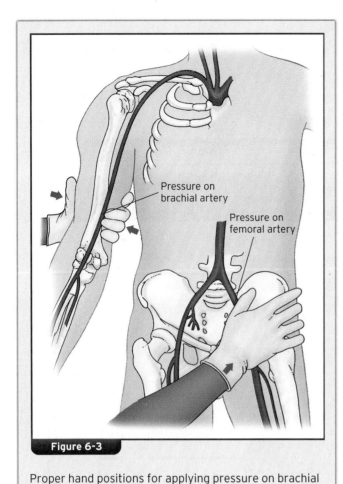

Figure 6-3

Proper hand positions for applying pressure on brachial and femoral arteries.

Pressure on brachial artery

Pressure on femoral artery

1. Rest the injured area.
2. Apply an ice or cold pack over the injury.
3. Apply an elastic bandage to compress the injured area.
4. Elevate an injured arm or leg, if it is not broken.

The RICE procedure is covered in more detail in Chapter 11.

To care for serious internal bleeding, follow these steps:

1. Call 9-1-1.
2. Care for shock by raising the victim's legs 6 to 12 inches, and cover the victim to maintain warmth. See Chapter 7 for more information on shock.
3. Expect vomiting. If vomiting occurs, roll the victim onto his or her side to allow drainage and to keep the airway clear.
4. Monitor breathing.

CAUTION

DO NOT give a victim anything to eat or drink. It could cause nausea and vomiting, which could result in inhaling foreign material into the lungs (aspiration). Food or liquids could cause complications during surgery if it is needed.

▶ Internal Bleeding

Internal bleeding occurs when the skin is not broken and blood is not seen. It can be difficult to detect, and it can be life threatening. A person with bleeding stomach ulcers, a lacerated liver, or a ruptured spleen may lose a large amount of blood into the abdomen with no outward sign of bleeding other than the presence of shock.

Recognizing Internal Bleeding

The signs of internal bleeding may appear quickly or take days to appear:

- Bruises or contusions of the skin
- Painful, tender area
- Vomiting or coughing up blood
- Stools that are black or contain bright red blood

Care for Internal Bleeding

For minor internal bleeding (such as a bruise on the leg from bumping into the corner of a table), follow the steps of the RICE procedure:

▶ Wound Care

A victim's wound should be cleaned to help prevent infection. Wound cleaning usually restarts bleeding by disturbing the clot, but it should be done anyway for shallow wounds. For severe bleeding or wounds with a high risk for infection (such as animal bites, deep puncture wounds, or dirty wounds), leave the pressure bandage in place until the victim can get medical care to clean the wound. To clean a shallow wound:

1. Wash inside the wound with soap and water.
2. Flush the wound with water from a faucet to provide sufficient quantity and pressure **Figure 6-4** . Run water directly into the wound and allow the water to run over the wound and out, thus carrying the dirty particles away from the wound. Flushing with water needs pressure to adequately cleanse the tissue. For a wound with a high risk for infection (eg, an animal bite, a very dirty or ragged wound, or a puncture), seek medical care for wound cleaning.
3. Remove small objects that don't flush out by irrigation with sterile tweezers.
4. If bleeding restarts, apply direct pressure.

Bleeding

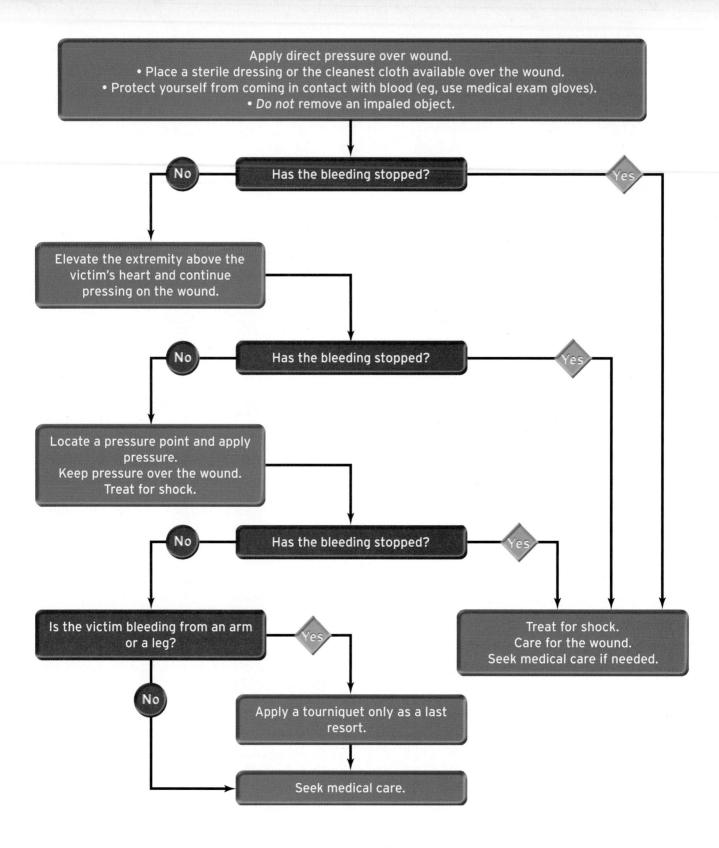

Apply direct pressure over wound.
- Place a sterile dressing or the cleanest cloth available over the wound.
- Protect yourself from coming in contact with blood (eg, use medical exam gloves).
- *Do not* remove an impaled object.

No — Has the bleeding stopped? — Yes

Elevate the extremity above the victim's heart and continue pressing on the wound.

No — Has the bleeding stopped? — Yes

Locate a pressure point and apply pressure.
Keep pressure over the wound.
Treat for shock.

No — Has the bleeding stopped? — Yes

Is the victim bleeding from an arm or a leg? — Yes

Treat for shock.
Care for the wound.
Seek medical care if needed.

No

Apply a tourniquet only as a last resort.

Seek medical care.

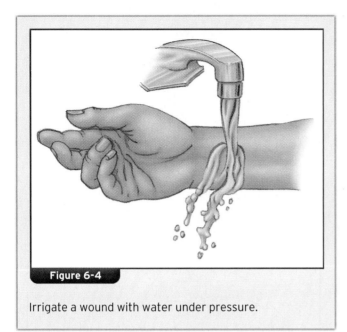

Figure 6-4

Irrigate a wound with water under pressure.

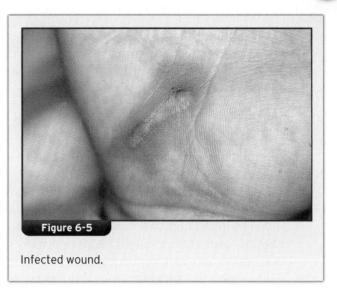

Figure 6-5

Infected wound.

5. Apply an antibiotic ointment such as Neosporin. Cover the area with a sterile and, if possible, non-stick dressing. To keep the dressing in place on an arm or a leg, use a roller bandage or tape; on other parts of the body, use tape.

6. Change the dressing daily, or more often if it gets wet or dirty. If a wound bleeds after a dressing has been applied and the dressing becomes stuck, leave it on as long as the wound is healing. Pulling the scab loose to change the dressing retards healing and increases the chance of infection. If a sticking dressing must be removed, soak it in warm water to help soften the scab and make removal easier.

CAUTION

DO NOT clean large, extremely dirty, or life-threatening wounds. Let hospital emergency department personnel do the cleaning.

DO NOT scrub a wound. Scrubbing a wound is debatable, and it can bruise the tissue.

DO NOT irrigate a wound with full-strength iodine preparations (eg, Betadine 10%) or isopropyl alcohol (70%). They kill body cells as well as bacteria and are painful. Also, some people are allergic to iodine.

DO NOT use hydrogen peroxide. It does not kill bacteria, it adversely affects capillary blood flow, and it extends wound healing.

DO NOT use antibiotic ointment on wounds that require sutures or on puncture wounds (the ointment may prevent drainage). Use an antibiotic ointment only on abrasions and shallow wounds.

▶ Wound Infection

Any wound, large or small, can become infected **Figure 6-5**. Once an infection begins, damage can be extensive, so prevention is the best way to avoid the problem. A wound should be cleaned using the procedures described above.

It is important to know how to recognize and treat an infected wound. The signs and symptoms of infection include:

- Swelling and redness around the wound
- A sensation of warmth
- Throbbing pain
- Pus discharge
- Fever
- Swelling of lymph nodes
- One or more red streaks leading from the wound toward the heart

FYI

Serious Sign of Infection

The appearance of one or more red streaks leading from the wound toward the heart is a serious sign that the infection is spreading and could cause death. If chills and fever develop, the infection has reached the circulatory system (known as *blood poisoning*). Seek medical care immediately.

Tetanus

The tetanus bacteria by itself does not cause tetanus. However, when it enters a wound that contains little oxygen (eg, a puncture wound), the bacteria can produce a powerful poisonous toxin. The toxin travels through the nervous system to the brain and the spinal cord. It then causes contractions of certain muscle groups (particularly in the jaw). There is no known antidote to the toxin after it enters the nervous system.

Tetanus can be prevented through vaccination. Everyone needs an initial series of vaccinations to prepare the immune system to defend against the toxin. A booster shot once every 5 to 10 years is sufficient to jog the immune system's memory.

The guidelines for tetanus immunization boosters are as follows:

- Anyone with a wound who has never been immunized against tetanus should be given a tetanus vaccine and booster immediately.
- A victim who was once immunized but has not received a tetanus booster within the last 10 years should receive a booster.
- A victim with a dirty wound who has not had a booster for over 5 years should receive a booster.
- Tetanus immunizations must be given within 72 hours of the injury to be effective.

▶ Special Wounds

This section addresses two special wounds: amputations and embedded (impaled) objects.

Amputations

The loss of a body part is a devastating injury that requires immediate medical care. To care for an amputation **Figure 6-6** :

1. Control the bleeding with direct pressure and elevate an extremity. Tourniquets are rarely needed and, if used, will destroy tissue, blood vessels, and nerves necessary for replantation.
2. Treat the victim for shock.
3. Recover the amputated part and, whenever possible, take it with the victim.
4. To care for the amputated body part:
   - Do not clean the amputated part.
   - Wrap the amputated part with a dry sterile gauze or other clean cloth.
   - Put the wrapped amputated part in a plastic bag or other waterproof container.
   - Keep the amputated part cool, but do not freeze. Place the bag or container with the wrapped part on a bed of ice.
5. Seek medical care immediately.

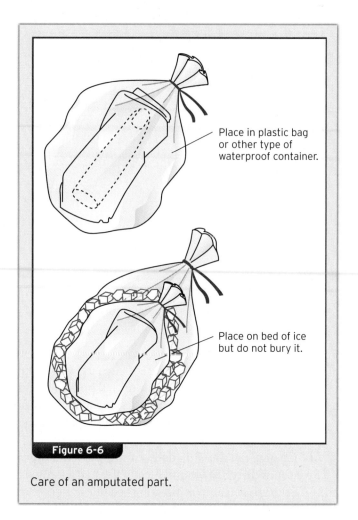

Place in plastic bag or other type of waterproof container.

Place on bed of ice but do not bury it.

Figure 6-6

Care of an amputated part.

FYI

Cooling Amputated Body Parts
Amputated body parts left uncooled for more than 6 hours have little chance of survival; 18 hours is probably the maximum time allowable for a part that has been cooled properly. Muscles without blood lose viability within 4 to 6 hours.

CAUTION

DO NOT wrap an amputated part in a wet dressing or cloth. Using a wet wrap on the part can cause water logging and tissue softening, which will make reattachment more difficult.

DO NOT bury an amputated part in ice-place it on ice. Reattaching frostbitten parts is usually unsuccessful.

Amputations

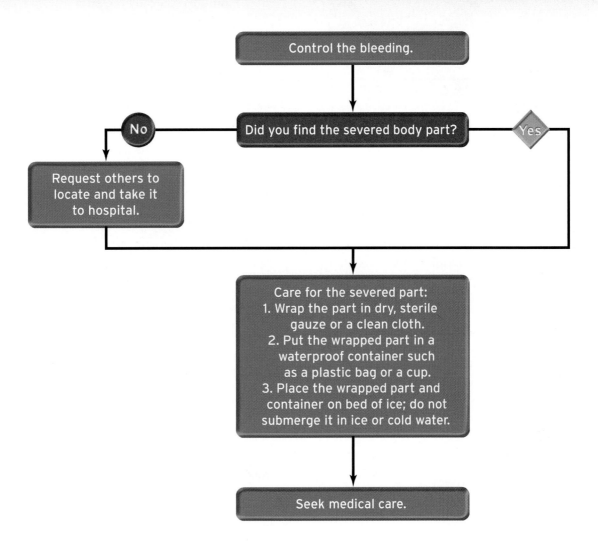

Control the bleeding.

Did you find the severed body part?

No — Request others to locate and take it to hospital.

Yes

Care for the severed part:
1. Wrap the part in dry, sterile gauze or a clean cloth.
2. Put the wrapped part in a waterproof container such as a plastic bag or a cup.
3. Place the wrapped part and container on bed of ice; do not submerge it in ice or cold water.

Seek medical care.

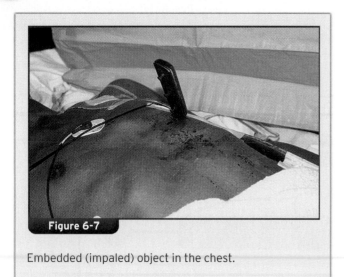

Figure 6-7

Embedded (impaled) object in the chest.

Embedded (Impaled) Objects

Objects such as glass, knives, and nails can be embedded (impaled) in the body **Figure 6-7**. To care for these wounds:

1. Expose the area. Remove or cut away clothing surrounding the injury.
2. Do not remove or move an impaled object. Movement of any kind could produce additional bleeding and tissue damage.
3. Control any bleeding with pressure around the impaled object. Do not press directly on the object.
4. Stabilize the object with bulky dressings or clean cloths around the object.
5. Shorten the object only if necessary.

▶ Wounds That Require Medical Care

It can be difficult to determine which wounds require a trip to the emergency department. These guidelines from the American College of Emergency Physicians identify which wounds need emergency medical care:

- Wounds that will not stop bleeding after 5 minutes of applying direct pressure
- Long or deep cuts that need stitches
- Cuts over a joint
- Cuts that may impair function of a body area, such as an eyelid or lip
- Cuts that remove all of the layers of the skin, such as those from slicing off the tip of a finger
- Cuts from an animal or human bite
- Cuts that have damaged or may have damaged underlying nerves, tendons, or joints
- Cuts over a possible broken bone

- Cuts caused by a crushing injury
- Cuts with an object embedded in them
- Cuts caused by metal object or a puncture wound

Call 9-1-1 immediately if:

- Bleeding from a cut does not slow during the first 15 minutes of steady pressure
- Signs of shock occur
- Breathing is difficult because of a cut to the neck or chest
- A deep cut to the abdomen causes moderate to severe pain
- A cut occurs to the eyeball
- A cut amputates or partially amputates an extremity

FYI

Sutures (Stitches)

If sutures are needed, they should be applied by a physician within 6 to 8 hours of the injury. Suturing wounds allows faster healing, reduces infection, and lessens scarring.

Some wounds do not usually require sutures:

- Wounds in which the skin's cut edges tend to fall together
- Shallow cuts less than 1 inch long

Rather than close a gaping wound with butterfly bandages, cover the wound with sterile gauze. Closing the wound might trap bacteria inside, resulting in an infection. In most cases, a physician can be reached in time for sutures to be made.

▶ Dressings and Bandages

First aid kits include dressings and bandages to be used when controlling bleeding and caring for wounds. A **dressing** is a covering that is placed directly over a wound to help absorb blood, prevent infection, and protect the wound from further injury. Dressings come in different shapes, sizes, and types. Dressings can be gauze pads (eg, 2- or 4-inch square or larger) used to cover larger wounds, or adhesive strips, such as Band-Aids, which are dressings combined with a bandage for small cuts or scrapes **Figure 6-8**.

A **bandage**, such as a roll of gauze, is often used to cover a dressing to keep it in place on the wound and to apply pressure to help control the bleeding. Like dressings, bandages also come in different shapes, sizes, and material **Figure 6-9**. Elastic bandages can be used to provide support and stability for an extremity or joint and to decrease swelling, but they are not usually used to cover wounds.

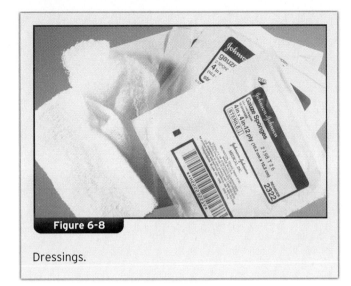

Figure 6-8

Dressings.

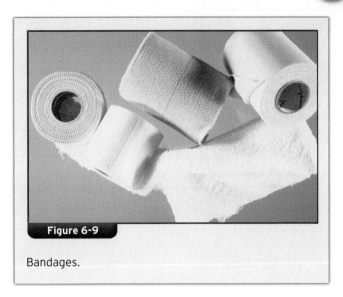

Figure 6-9

Bandages.

When commercial bandages are unavailable, improvise bandages from neckties, bandannas, or strips of cloth torn from a sheet or other similar material.

When applying a bandage, do not apply it so tightly that it restricts blood circulation. The signs that a bandage is too tight are as follows:

- Blue tinge to the fingernails or toenails
- Blue or pale skin
- Tingling or loss of sensation
- Coldness of the extremity

▶ Bleeding

What to Look For	What to Do
External bleeding • Blood coming from an open wound	1. Protect against blood contact. 2. Place sterile dressing over wound and apply pressure. 3. Elevate the injured area if possible. 4. Apply a pressure bandage. 5. If bleeding cannot be controlled, apply pressure to a pressure point.

Internal bleeding
• Bruising
• Painful, tender area
• Vomiting or coughing up blood
• Stool that is black or contains bright red blood
	Minor internal bleeding:
	1. Use RICE procedures:
	  R = Rest
	  I = Ice or cold pack
	  C = Compress the area with elastic bandage
	  E = Elevate the injured extremity
	
	Serious internal bleeding:
	1. Call 9-1-1.
	2. Care for shock.
	3. If vomiting occurs, roll the victim onto side.

▶ Wounds

What to Look For	What to Do
Wound care	1. Wash with soap and water. 2. Flush with running water under pressure. 3. Remove remaining small object(s). 4. If the bleeding restarts, apply pressure on wound. 5. Apply antibiotic ointment. 6. Cover with sterile or clean dressing. 7. For wounds with a high risk for infection, seek medical care for cleaning, possible tetanus booster, and closing.
Wound infection • Swelling and redness around the wound • Sensation of warmth • Throbbing pain • Pus discharge • Fever • Swelling of lymph nodes • Red streaks leading from the wound toward the heart	1. Seek medical care. A physician may allow: 1. Soaking the wound in warm water or applying warm, wet packs. 2. Applying antibiotic ointment. 3. Changing the dressings daily.
Amputation • Loss of a body part	1. Call 9-1-1. 2. Control bleeding. 3. Care for shock. 4. Recover amputated part(s) and wrap in sterile or clean dressing. 5. Place wrapped part(s) in a plastic bag or waterproof container. 6. Keep part(s) cool.
Embedded (impaled) object • Object remains in wound • Call 9-1-1.	1. Do not remove object. 2. Control bleeding with pressure around the object. 3. Stabilize the object with bulky dressings or clean cloths.

▶ Ready for Review

- External bleeding occurs when blood can be seen coming from an open wound.
- The three types of external bleeding are (1) arterial, (2) venous, and (3) capillary.
- The types of open wounds are (1) abrasion, (2) laceration, (3) incision, (4) puncture, (5) avulsion, and (6) amputation.
- Proper first aid of an impaled object requires that the object be stabilized because significant internal damage can occur.
- Internal bleeding is difficult to detect and can be life threatening.
- Care for shallow wounds by (1) washing with soap and water, (2) flushing with water under pressure, (3) applying antibiotic ointment, (4) covering with a dressing.
- Care for a wound with a high risk for infection (eg, animal bite, puncture wound, dirty wound) should be done by trained medical personnel.
- A tetanus vaccination can prevent tetanus.
- In many cases, an amputated extremity can be successfully replanted if the part is properly preserved.

▶ Vital Vocabulary

arterial bleeding Blood spurts (up to several feet) from the wound.

bandage Used to cover a dressing to keep it in place and to apply pressure to help control bleeding.

capillary bleeding The most common type of bleeding, blood oozes from capillaries.

dressing Covering that is placed directly over wound to help absorb blood, prevent infection and protect the wound.

hemorrhage A large amount of bleeding in a short time.

venous bleeding Blood from a vein flows steadily or gushes.

▶ Assessment in Action

A 25-year-old construction worker has been badly cut on his thigh by a circular power saw. The cut is approximately 5 inches long, and blood is spurting from the wound.
Directions: Circle *Yes* if you agree with the statement and *No* if you disagree.

Yes No 1. This victim is experiencing venous bleeding.
Yes No 2. You should wash this wound with soap and water.
Yes No 3. Direct pressure should stop the bleeding.
Yes No 4. The type of bleeding experienced by this man is the most common type.

Answers: 1. No; 2. No; 3. Yes; 4. No

▶ Check Your Knowledge

Directions: Circle *Yes* if you agree with the statement and *No* if you disagree.

Yes No 1. Most cases of bleeding require more than direct pressure to stop the bleeding.
Yes No 2. Elevating an arm or leg alone will not control bleeding and must be used in combination with direct pressure over the wound.
Yes No 3. If direct pressure and elevation fail to control bleeding, the next step would be to use a tourniquet.
Yes No 4. Applying pressure to pressure points in the arms or legs is often needed to control bleeding.
Yes No 5. Wash shallow wounds with soapy water.
Yes No 6. Irrigating a wound with water needs pressure.
Yes No 7. Wounds with a high risk for infection (eg, animal bites, dirty wounds) require medical care for proper wound cleaning.
Yes No 8. Antibiotic ointment can be applied to any wound.
Yes No 9. Recover any amputated part, regardless of size, and take it with the victim to the nearest hospital.
Yes No 10. Keep an amputated part packed (buried) in ice.

Answers: 1. No; 2. Yes; 3. No; 4. No; 5. Yes; 6. Yes; 7. Yes; 8. No; 9. Yes; 10. No

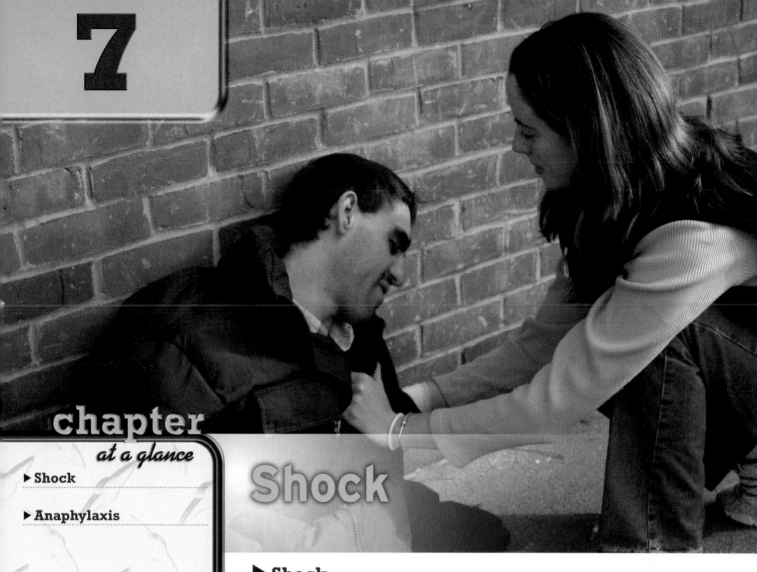

chapter
at a glance

▶ Shock

▶ Anaphylaxis

Shock

▶ Shock

<u>Shock</u> occurs when the body's tissues do not receive enough oxygenated blood. Because every injury affects the circulatory system to some degree, first aiders should automatically treat injured victims for shock.

To understand shock, think of the circulatory system as having three components: a working pump (the heart), a network of pipes (the blood vessels), and an adequate amount of fluid (the blood) pumped through the pipes. Damage to any of these components can deprive tissues of blood and produce the condition known as shock. These three parts can be referred to as the *perfusion triangle* **Figure 7-1** .

Shock can be classified as one of three types according to which component fails:

- *Pump failure.* The heart cannot pump sufficient blood. For example, a major heart attack can damage the heart muscle so the heart cannot squeeze, and therefore cannot push blood through the blood vessels.
- *Fluid loss.* A significant amount of fluid, usually blood, is lost from the system.
- *Pipe failure.* Blood vessels (pipes) enlarge, and the blood supply is insufficient to fill them. This can result when the nervous system is damaged, such as with a spinal injury or drug overdose.

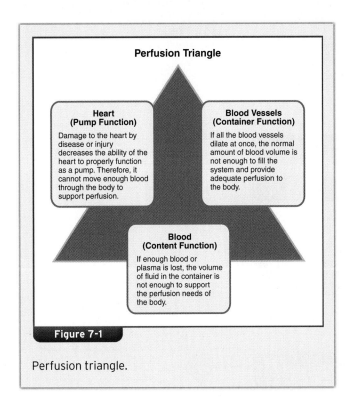

Figure 7-1

Perfusion triangle.

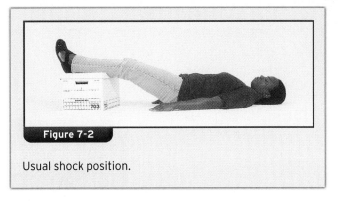

Figure 7-2

Usual shock position.

Recognizing Shock

The signs of shock include the following:

- Altered mental status: anxiety, restlessness, agitation, confusion
- Pale, cold, and clammy skin, lips, and nail beds
- Nausea and vomiting
- Rapid breathing and pulse
- Unresponsiveness when shock is severe

Care for Shock

Even if an injured victim does not have signs or symptoms of shock, first aiders should treat for shock:

1. Treat life-threatening injuries and other severe injuries.
2. Lay the victim on his or her back.
3. Raise the victim's legs 6 to 12 inches. Raising the legs allows the blood to drain from the legs back to the heart **Figure 7-2**. Other positions may be used in shock when other conditions are present **Figure 7-3 A-D**.
4. Prevent body heat loss by putting blankets and coats under and over the victim.

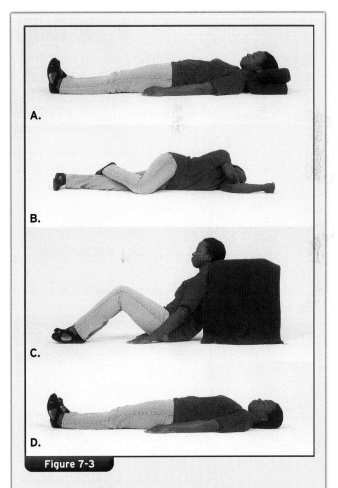

Figure 7-3

A. For a victim with a head injury, elevate the head (if spinal injury is not suspected). **B.** Position an unresponsive or stroke victim in the recovery position. **C.** Use a half-sitting position for victims with breathing difficulties, chest injuries, or a heart attack. **D.** Keep the victim flat if a spinal injury or leg fracture is suspected.

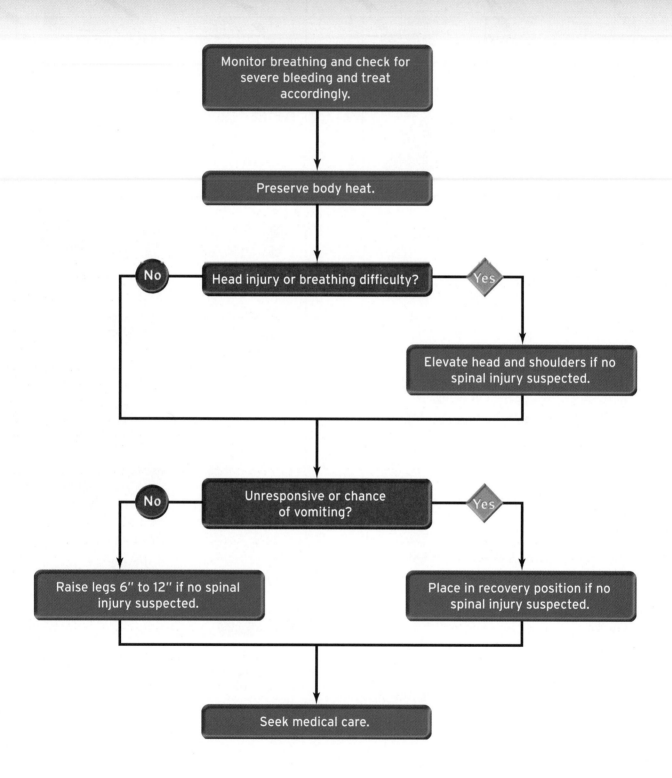

▶ Anaphylaxis

A powerful reaction to substances eaten or injected can occur within minutes or even seconds. This reaction, called **anaphylaxis**, can cause death if it is not treated immediately.

Well-known causes of anaphylaxis include:

- Medications (penicillin and related drugs, aspirin, sulfa drugs)
- Food and food additives (shellfish, nuts, eggs, monosodium glutamate, nitrates, nitrites)
- Insect stings (honeybee, yellow jacket, wasp, hornet, fire ant)
- Plant pollen

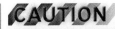

DO NOT mistake anaphylaxis for other reactions such as hyperventilation, anxiety attacks, alcohol intoxication, or low blood sugar.

Recognizing Anaphylaxis

Anaphylaxis typically comes on within minutes of exposure to the offending substance, peaks in 15 to 30 minutes, and may be over within hours. The most common signs of anaphylaxis include:

- Breathing difficulty—shortness of breath and wheezing
- Skin reaction—itching or burning skin, especially over the face and upper part of the chest, with rash or hives
- Swelling of the tongue, mouth, or throat

Other signs of anaphylaxis are:

- Sneezing, coughing
- Tightness in the chest
- Blueness around lips and mouth
- Dizziness
- Nausea and vomiting

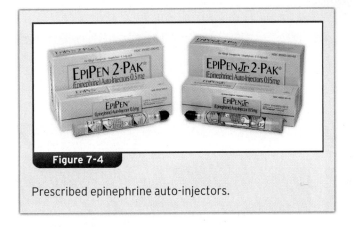

Figure 7-4

Prescribed epinephrine auto-injectors.

Care for Anaphylaxis

To care for anaphylaxis:

1. Call 9-1-1 immediately.
2. Monitor breathing and, if necessary, give CPR.
3. Determine if the victim has medication for allergic reactions. If the victim has a prescribed **epinephrine auto-injector** `Figure 7-4`, help the victim use it. If you are assisting with or using an auto-injector, follow the steps in `Skill Drill 7-1`.
   a. Remove the safety cap. The auto-injector is now ready for use (**Step ❶**).
   b. Support the victim's thigh and place the black tip of the auto-injector lightly against the outer thigh.
   c. Using a quick motion, push the auto-injector firmly against the thigh and hold it in place for several seconds (**Step ❷**). This will inject the medication.
   d. Remove the auto-injector from the thigh. Carefully reinsert the used auto-injector, needle first, into the carrying tube (**Step ❸**). A small amount of medication will remain in the device, but the device cannot be reused.
4. Give an antihistamine (such as Benadryl)—it is not life saving, because it takes too long to work (20 minutes), but it can prevent later reactions.
5. Keep a responsive victim sitting up to help breathing. Place an unresponsive breathing victim on his or her side.

skill drill

7-1   Using an Epinephrine Auto-Injector

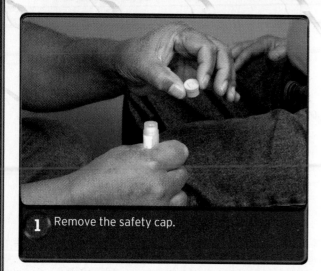

1 Remove the safety cap.

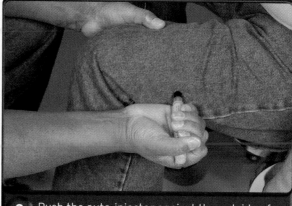

2 Push the auto-injector against the outside of the thigh and hold in place for several seconds.

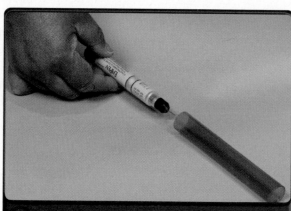

3 Re-insert the used auto-injector, needle first, into the carrying tube.

▶ Shock and Anaphylaxis

What to Look For

What to Look For | What to Do

Shock
- Altered mental status (anxiety, restlessness)
- Pale, cold, and clammy skin, lips, and nail beds
- Nausea and vomiting
- Rapid breathing

1. Place the victim on his or her back and raise the legs 6 to 12 inches. Other positions are used for other conditions.
2. Place blankets under and over the victim to keep the victim warm.

Anaphylaxis
- Breathing difficulty
- Skin reaction
- Swelling of the tongue, mouth, or throat
- Sneezing, coughing
- Tightness in the chest
- Blueness around lips and mouth
- Dizziness
- Nausea and vomiting

1. Call 9-1-1.
2. Determine if victim has a prescribed epinephrine auto-injector and help the victim use it.
3. Keep a responsive victim sitting up to help breathing. Place an unresponsive victim on his or her side.

prep kit

▶ Ready for Review

- Shock is a failure of the cardiovascular system in which blood circulation decreases and blood is distributed unevenly throughout the body.
- The damage caused by shock depends on which body part is deprived of oxygen and for how long.
- Causes of shock can be both cardiovascular and noncardiovascular.
- Anaphylaxis occurs when the immune system reacts violently to a substance to which it has already been sensitized.
- First aiders should automatically treat victims for shock.

▶ Vital Vocabulary

anaphylaxis A life-threatening allergic reaction.

epinephrine auto-injector Prescribed device used to administer an emergency dose of epinephrine to a victim experiencing anaphylaxis.

shock Inadequate tissue oxygenation resulting from serious injury or illness.

▶ Assessment in Action

Your neighbor was working in her garden on a warm summer day. She unintentionally disturbed a nest of yellow jackets and was stung several times on her face and neck. She has begun coughing and wheezing. She complains that she is dizzy and having difficulty breathing. You notice that her face is swelling.

Directions: Circle *Yes* if you agree with the statement and *No* if you disagree.

Yes   No   1. Breathing difficulty and swelling may be signs of a severe allergic reaction.

Yes   No   2. Ask the victim if he or she has prescribed epinephrine.

Yes   No   3. The condition this victim is experiencing is life threatening, and medical care is needed.

Yes   No   4. Place this victim in the usual shock position—lying down with the legs raised.

Answers: 1. Yes; 2. Yes; 3. Yes; 4. No

▶ Check Your Knowledge

Directions: Circle *Yes* if you agree with the statement and *No* if you disagree.

Yes   No   1. Most victims of shock should be placed flat on their backs.

Yes   No   2. Give the victim something to drink.

Yes   No   3. Prevent body heat loss by putting blankets under and over the victim.

Yes   No   4. A shock victim with head injuries should be placed on his or her side.

Yes   No   5. A shock victim with breathing difficulty or chest injury should be placed on his or her back with the legs raised.

Yes   No   6. Anaphylaxis is another form of fainting.

Yes   No   7. Anaphylaxis can kill.

Yes   No   8. Ask the victim of anaphylaxis if he or she has a doctor prescribed epinephrine injector.

Yes   No   9. Treat severely injured victims for shock even if there are no signs of it.

Yes   No   10. An epinephrine auto-injector requires a doctor's prescription.

Answers: 1. No; 2. No; 3. Yes; 4. No; 5. No; 6. No; 7. Yes; 8. Yes; 9. Yes; 10. Yes

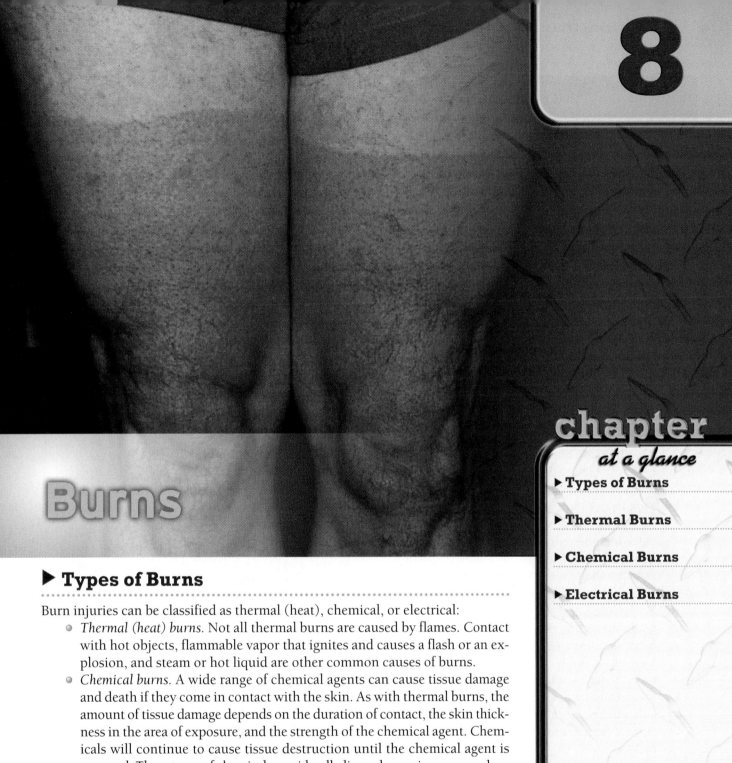

Burns

▶ Types of Burns

Burn injuries can be classified as thermal (heat), chemical, or electrical:

- *Thermal (heat) burns.* Not all thermal burns are caused by flames. Contact with hot objects, flammable vapor that ignites and causes a flash or an explosion, and steam or hot liquid are other common causes of burns.
- *Chemical burns.* A wide range of chemical agents can cause tissue damage and death if they come in contact with the skin. As with thermal burns, the amount of tissue damage depends on the duration of contact, the skin thickness in the area of exposure, and the strength of the chemical agent. Chemicals will continue to cause tissue destruction until the chemical agent is removed. Three types of chemicals—acids, alkalis, and organic compounds—are responsible for most chemical burns.
- *Electrical burns.* The severity of an injury from contact with electrical current depends on the type of current (direct or alternating), the voltage, the area of the body exposed, and the duration of contact.

▶ Thermal Burns

Evaluate a thermal burn using the following steps. These steps form the basis for treatment of thermal burns.

1. Determine the depth (degree) of the burn. Making an assessment of burn depth will help you decide whether to seek medical care for the victim.

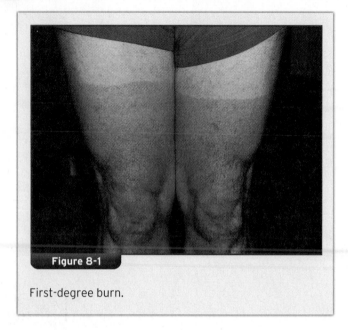

Figure 8-1

First-degree burn.

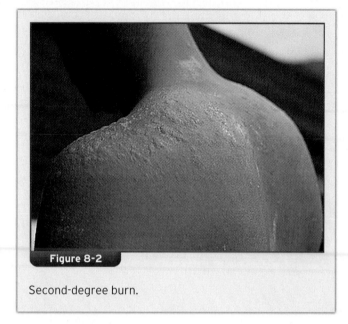

Figure 8-2

Second-degree burn.

You should be aware that it can be difficult to tell a burn's depth because the destruction varies within the same burn. Even experienced physicians may not know the true depth for several days after the burn.

- **First-degree (superficial) burns** affect the skin's outer layer (epidermis) **Figure 8-1** . Characteristics include redness, mild swelling, tenderness, and pain. Healing occurs without scarring, usually within a week. The outer edges of deeper burns often are first-degree burns.

- **Second-degree (partial-thickness) burns** extend through the entire outer layer and into the inner skin layer **Figure 8-2** . Blisters, swelling, weeping of fluids, and pain characterize these burns, because the capillary blood vessels in the dermis are damaged and give up fluid into surrounding tissues. Intact blisters provide a sterile, waterproof covering. Once a blister breaks, a weeping wound results and the risk of infection increases.

- **Third-degree (full-thickness) burns** are severe burns that penetrate all the skin layers, into the underlying fat and muscle **Figure 8-3** . The skin looks leathery, waxy, or pearly gray and sometimes charred. There is a dry appearance, because capillary blood vessels have been destroyed and no more fluid is brought to the area. The skin does not blanch after being pressed because the area is dead. The victim feels no pain from a third-degree burn because the nerve endings have been damaged or destroyed. Any pain that

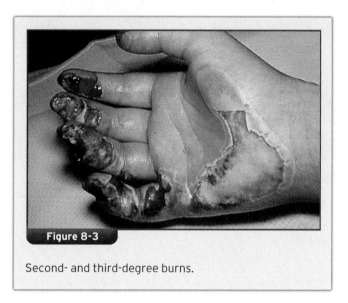

Figure 8-3

Second- and third-degree burns.

is felt is from surrounding burns of lesser degrees. Medical care for a third-degree burn involves removing the dead tissue and often a skin graft to heal properly.

FYI

Respiratory Injuries
Respiratory damage may result from breathing heat or the products of combustion; from being burned by a flame while in a closed space; or from being in an explosion. Swelling occurs in 2 to 24 hours, restricting or even completely shutting off the airway so that air cannot reach the lungs. All respiratory injuries must receive medical care.

2. Determine the extent of the burn. This means estimating how much body surface area the burn covers. A rough guide known as the *Rule of Nines* assigns a percentage value to each part of an adult's body. The entire head is 9%, one complete arm is 9%, the front torso is 18%, the complete back is 18%, and each leg is 18%. The Rule of Nines must be modified to take into account the different proportions of a small child. In small children and infants, the head accounts for 18% and each leg is 14%. For small or scattered burns, use the *Rule of the Palm*. The victim's hand, excluding the fingers and the thumb, represents about 1% of his or her total body surface ⬛Figure 8-4⬛. Estimate the unburned area in number of hands.

CAUTION

DO NOT remove clothing stuck to the skin–pulling will further damage the skin.

DO NOT forget to remove jewelry as soon as possible– swelling could make jewelry difficult to remove later.

3. Determine what parts of the body are burned. Burns on the face, hands, feet, and genitals are more severe than on other body parts. A circumferential burn (one that goes around a finger, toe, arm, leg, neck, or chest) is considered more severe than a noncircumferential one because it can have constriction and tourniquet effects on circu-

lation and, in some cases, breathing. All these burns require medical care.

4. Determine if other injuries or preexisting medical problems exist or if the victim is elderly (over 55) or very young (under five). A medical problem or belonging to one of those age groups increases a burn's severity.

5. Determine the burn's severity ⬛Table 8-1⬛. This forms the basis for how to treat the burned victim. Most burns are minor, occur at home, and can be managed outside a medical setting. Seek medical care for all moderate and severe burns, as classified by the American Burn Association (ABA).

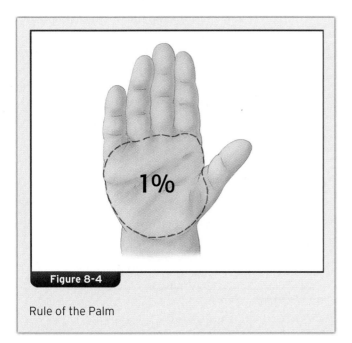

Figure 8-4

Rule of the Palm

Table 8-1   Burn Severity

Minor Burns
- First-degree burn covering less than 50% BSA* in adults (face, hands, feet, and genitals not burned)
- Second-degree burn covering less than 15% BSA in adults
- Second-degree burn covering less than 10% BSA in children/elderly persons
- Third-degree burn covering less than 2% BSA in adults (face, hands, feet, or genitals not burned)

Moderate Burns
- First-degree burn covering more than 50% BSA in adults
- Second-degree burn covering 15% to 30% BSA in adults
- Second-degree burn covering 10% to 20% BSA in children/elderly persons
- Third-degree burn covering 2% to 10% BSA in adults (face, hands, or feet not burned)

Critical Burns
- First-degree burn covering more than 70% BSA
- Second-degree burn covering more than 30% BSA in adults
- Second-degree burn covering more than 20% BSA in children/elderly persons
- Third-degree burn covering more than 10% BSA in adults
- Third-degree burn covering more than 2% BSA in children/elderly persons or any part of the face, hands, feet, or genitals
- Also most inhalation injuries, electrical injuries, and burns accompanied by major trauma or significant preexisting conditions

*BSA = body surface area

Care for Thermal Burns

Burn care aims to reduce pain, protect against infection, and prevent evaporation. Seek medical care if any of the following conditions apply:

- The victim is under 5 or over 55 years of age.
- The victim has difficulty breathing.
- Other injuries exist.
- An electrical injury exists.
- The face, hands, feet, or genitals are burned.
- Child abuse is suspected.
- The surface area of a second-degree burn is greater than 15% of the body surface area.
- The burn is third-degree.

Care of First-Degree Burns

1. Immerse the burned area in cold water or apply a wet, cold cloth to reduce pain. Apply cold until the part is pain free both in and out of the water (usually in 10 minutes, but it may take up to 45 minutes) **Figure 8-5**. Cold also stops the burn from progressing into deeper tissue. If cold water is unavailable, use any clean cold liquid to reduce the temperature of the burned skin.
2. Give ibuprofen to relieve pain and inflammation. Give children acetaminophen.
3. After the burn cools, apply an aloe vera gel or an inexpensive skin moisturizer lotion to keep the

skin moistened and to reduce itching and peeling. Aloe vera has antimicrobial properties and is an effective analgesic.

4. Keep a burned arm or leg elevated.

CAUTION

DO NOT apply cold to more than 20% of an adult's body surface (10% for children); widespread cooling can cause hypothermia. Burn victims lose large amounts of heat and water.

DO NOT apply salve, ointment, grease, butter, cream, spray, home remedy, or any other coating on a burn. Such coatings are unsterile and can lead to infection. They also can seal in heat, causing further damage.

Care of Small Second-Degree Burns (<20% BSA)

1. Follow steps 1 and 2 of first-degree burn care.
2. After the burn cools, apply a thin layer of antibiotic ointment such as Bacitracin. Topical antibiotic therapy does not sterilize a wound, but it does decrease the number of bacteria to a level that can be controlled by the body's defense mechanisms and prevents the entrance of bacteria.
3. Cover the burn with a dry, nonstick, sterile dressing or a clean cloth. Covering the burn reduces the amount of pain by keeping air from the exposed nerve endings. The main purpose of a dressing over a burn is to keep the burn clean, prevent moisture loss through evaporation, and reduce pain. If toes or fingers have been burned, place dry dressings between them.
4. Have the victim drink water as tolerated without becoming nauseous.

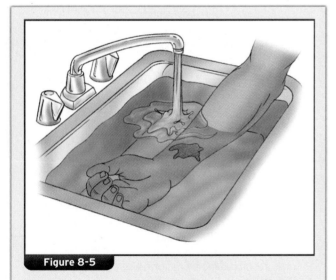

Figure 8-5

Cool first-degree and small second-degree burns until the pain is relieved. Cooling usually takes at least 10 minutes.

CAUTION

DO NOT cool more than 20% of an adult's body surface area (10% for a child), except to extinguish flames.

DO NOT break any blisters. Intact blisters serve as excellent burn dressings. Cover a ruptured blister with Bacitracin ointment and a dry, sterile dressing.

Thermal Burns

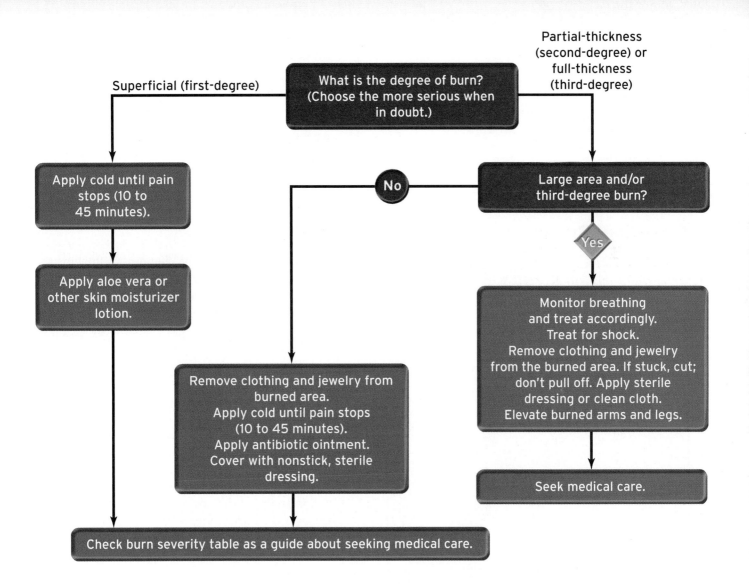

Care of Large Second-Degree Burns (>20% BSA)

Do not apply cold to a large second-degree burn, because it may cause hypothermia. To care for a second-degree burn, follow these steps:

1. Follow steps 3 and 4 of small second-degree burn care (<20% BSA).
2. Seek medical care.

Care of Third-Degree Burns

1. Cover the burn with a dry, nonstick, sterile dressing or a clean cloth.
2. Treat the victim for shock by elevating the legs and keeping the victim warm with a clean sheet or blanket.
3. Seek medical care.

▶ Chemical Burns

A chemical burn is the result of a caustic or corrosive substance touching the skin **Figure 8-6**. Because chemicals continue to "burn" as long as they are in contact with the skin, they should be removed from the victim as rapidly as possible.

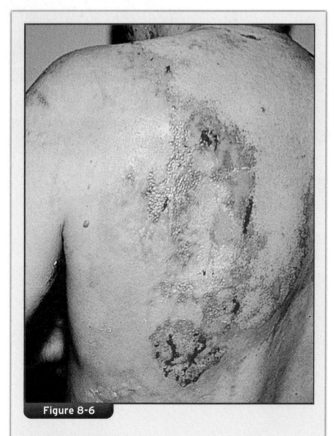

Figure 8-6

Chemical burn from sulfuric acid.

First aid is the same for all chemical burns, except a few specific ones for which a chemical neutralizer has to be used. Alkalis such as drain cleaners cause more serious burns than acids such as battery acid, because they penetrate deeper and remain active longer. Organic compounds such as petroleum products are also capable of burning.

CAUTION

DO NOT apply water under high pressure—it will drive the chemical deeper into the tissue.

DO NOT try to neutralize a chemical even if you know which chemical is involved—heat may be produced, resulting in more damage. Some product labels for neutralizing may be wrong. Save the container or the label for the chemical's name.

Care for Chemical Burns

1. Immediately remove the chemical by flushing the area with water **Figure 8-7A, B**. If available, use a hose or a shower. Brush dry powder chemicals from the skin before flushing, unless large amounts of water are immediately available **Figure 8-8**. Water may activate a dry chemical and cause more damage to the skin. Take precautions to protect yourself from exposure to the chemical.
2. Remove the victim's contaminated clothing and jewelry while flushing with water. Clothing can hold chemicals, allowing them to continue to burn as long as they are in contact with the skin.
3. Flush for 20 minutes or longer. Washing with large amounts of water dilutes the chemical concentration and washes it away.
4. Cover the burned area with a dry, sterile dressing or, for large areas, a clean cloth such as a pillowcase.
5. Seek medical care immediately for all chemical burns.

▶ Electrical Burns

Even a mild electrical shock can cause serious internal injuries. A current of 1,000 volts or more is considered high voltage, but even the 110 volts found in ordinary household current can be deadly.

There are three types of electrical injuries: thermal burn (flame), arc burn (flash), and true electrical injury (contact). A *thermal burn* (flame) results when clothing or objects in direct contact with the skin are ignited by an electrical current. These injuries are caused by the flames produced by the electrical current and not by the passage of the electrical current or arc.

Chemical Burns

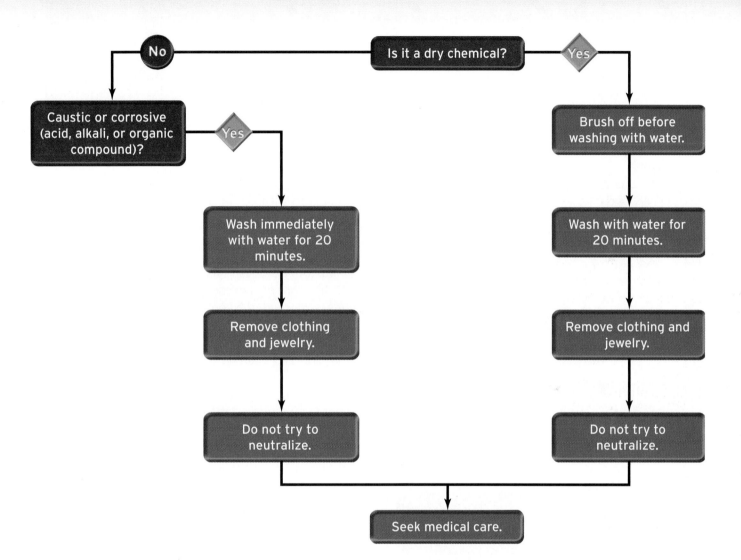

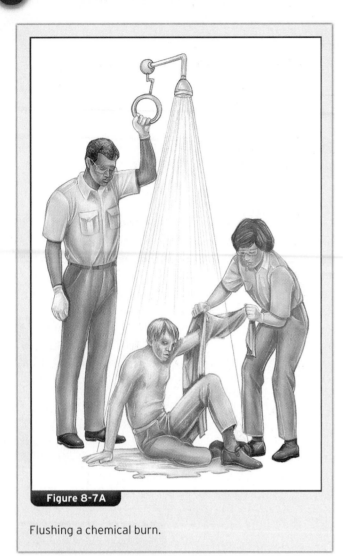

Figure 8-7A

Flushing a chemical burn.

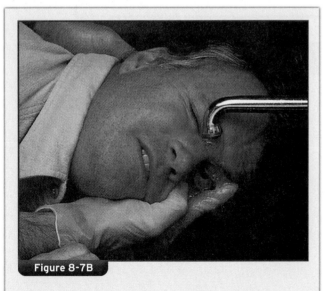

Figure 8-7B

Flush a chemical in an eye from the bridge of the nose outward.

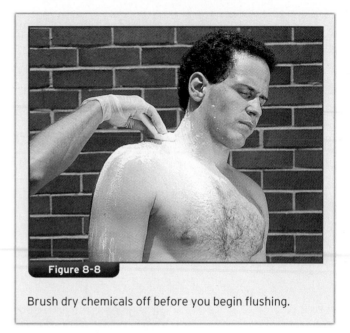

Figure 8-8

Brush dry chemicals off before you begin flushing.

An *arc burn* (flash) occurs when electricity jumps, or arcs, from one spot to another. The electrical current does not pass through the body. Although the duration of the flash may be brief, it usually causes extensive superficial injuries.

A *true electrical injury* (contact) happens when an electric current truly passes through the body. This type of injury is characterized by an entrance wound and an exit wound **Figure 8-9A, B** . The important factor in this type of injury is that the surface injury may be just the tip of the iceberg. High-voltage electrical currents passing through the body may disrupt the normal heart rhythm and cause cardiac arrest, burns, and other injuries.

FYI

Electric Shock

During an electric shock, electricity enters the body at the point of contact and travels along the path of least resistance (nerves and blood vessels). The major damage occurs inside the body—the outside burn may appear small. Usually, the electricity exits where the body touches a surface or comes in contact with a ground (eg, a metal object). Sometimes, a victim has more than one exit site.

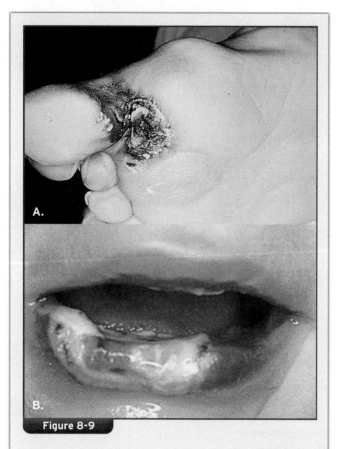

Figure 8-9

Electrical burns. **A.** Exit wound on a toe. **B.** Electrical burn caused by chewing through an electrical cord.

Care for Electrical Burns

1. Make sure the area is safe. Unplug, disconnect, or turn off the power. If that is not possible, call the power company or 9-1-1 for help.
2. Monitor breathing.
3. If the victim fell, check for a spinal injury.
4. Treat the victim for shock.
5. Seek medical care immediately. Electrical injuries usually require burn center care.

Contact with a Power Line (Outdoors)

If the electric shock is from contact with a downed power line, the power *must* be turned off before a rescuer approaches anyone who may be in contact with the wire. If you can safely reach the victim, do not attempt to move any wires, even with wooden poles, tools with wood handles, or tree branches. Even objects that seem to be insulating, such as dry wood, can conduct lethal amounts of energy to a rescuer. Do not attempt to move downed wires at all unless you are trained and are equipped with tools that can handle the high voltage. Wait until trained personnel with the proper equipment can cut the wires or disconnect them. Prevent bystanders from entering the danger area.

Contact Inside Buildings

Most electrical burns that occur indoors are caused by faulty electrical equipment or careless use of electrical appliances. Turn off the electricity at the circuit breaker, fuse box, or outside switch box or unplug the appliance if the plug is undamaged. Do not touch the appliance or the victim until the current is off. Once there is no danger to rescuers, first aid can begin.

▶ Thermal (Heat) Burns

What to Look For | What to Do

First-degree burn
- Redness
- Mild swelling
- Pain

1. Cool the burn with cold water.
2. Apply aloe vera gel or a skin moisturizer.
3. If available, give an over-the-counter pain medication.

Second-degree burn
- Blisters
- Swelling
- Pain
- Weeping of fluid

If burn is small (<20% BSA):
1. Cool the burn with cold water.
2. Apply antibiotic ointment.
3. Cover with a dry, nonstick, sterile dressing.
4. If available, give an over-the-counter pain medication.
If burn is large (>20% BSA):
1. Follow steps for a third-degree burn.

Third-degree burns
- Dry, leathery skin
- Gray or charred skin

1. Monitor breathing and provide care as needed.
2. Cover burn with a dry, nonstick, sterile or clean dressing.
3. Care for shock.
4. Seek medical care.

▶ Chemical Burns

What to Look For | What to Do

- Stinging pain

1. Brush dry powder chemicals off skin.
2. Flush with a large amount of water for 20 minutes.
3. Remove victim's contaminated clothing and jewelry while flushing.
4. Cover area with a dry, sterile or clean dressing.
5. Seek medical care.

▶ Electrical Burns

What to Look For | What to Do

- Possible third-degree burn with entrance and exit wounds

1. Safety first! Unplug, disconnect, or turn off the electricity.
2. Open the airway, check breathing, and provide care as needed.
3. Care for burns as you would a third-degree burn.
4. Call 9-1-1.

► Ready for Review

- Burn injuries can be classified as thermal, chemical, or electrical.
- The depth of a burn can be classified as first, second, and third degree.
- The extent of a burn or body surface area affected can be determined by either the Rule of Nines or the Rule of the Palm.
- Burns on the face, hands, feet, and genitals are more severe than those on other body parts.
- Cold water should be used on first- and small second-degree burns, but not on more extensive second-degree or third-degree burns.
- After the burn has cooled, aloe vera or a skin moisturizer lotion can be placed on first-degree and small second-degree burns. Apply an antibiotic ointment such as Bacitracin on large second-degree burns.
- Cover large second-degree and third-degree burns with a dressing and seek medical care.
- Chemical burns should be flushed with water for 20 minutes.
- Electrical burns require medical care.

► Vital Vocabulary

first-degree (superficial) burn Affects the skin's outer layer (epidermis).

second-degree (partial-thickness) burn Extends through the entire outer layer and into the inner skin layer.

third-degree (full-thickness) burn Severe burn that penetrates all the skin layers, into the underlying fat and muscle.

► Assessment in Action

Tracy is boiling water to make hot chocolate in the office kitchen. She reaches across the stove for a cup. The sleeve of her blouse touches the flame of the gas burner and ignites, sending fire racing up her arm. Her screams bring you and others racing into the kitchen. You put out the flames and remove any burned clothing. You see that her skin is red and blistered on one side of her arm.

Directions: Circle *Yes* if you agree with the statement and *No* if you disagree.

Yes   No   **1.** Blisters are one of the best signs of a second-degree burn.

Yes   No   **2.** Treat the burned area with cold water.

Yes   No   **3.** Once the burn is cooled, apply an antibiotic ointment over the affected area.

Yes   No   **4.** This victim needs medical care.

Answers: **1.** Yes; **2.** Yes; **3.** Yes; **4.** No

► Check Your Knowledge

Directions: Circle *Yes* if you agree with the statement and *No* if you disagree.

Yes   No   **1.** Relieve pain and tissue damage from a burn by holding the part in a sink filled with running cold water.

Yes   No   **2.** Pain and inflammation can be relieved with ibuprofen.

Yes   No   **3.** After a first-degree burn has been cooled, a layer of aloe vera gel can be applied on the affected area.

Yes   No   **4.** Butter can be effective on first- and second-degree burns.

Yes   No   **5.** When washing chemicals off the body, flush with water for at least 5 minutes.

Yes   No   **6.** When washing chemicals off the body, use high pressure water.

Yes   No   **7.** Do not try to neutralize a chemical, because more damage may result.

Yes   No   **8.** The Rule of the Palm is used to determine the size or extent of a burn.

Yes   No   **9.** If an electrocuted victim is in contact with an outdoor electrical wire, try to move it with a wooden pole or handle.

Yes   No   **10.** If an electrocuted victim is inside a building, turn off electricity at the fuse box, circuit-breaker, outside switch box, or unplug the appliance before approaching him or her.

Answers: **1.** Yes; **2.** Yes; **3.** Yes; **4.** No; **5.** No; **6.** No; **7.** Yes; **8.** Yes; **9.** No; **10.** Yes

9

Head and Spinal Injuries

Head Injuries

Head injury is a broadly used term. Different types of head injuries include scalp wounds, skull fractures, and brain injuries. Neck and spine injuries can be present in head-injured victims.

▶ Scalp Wounds

A bleeding scalp wound does not affect the blood supply to the brain. The brain obtains its blood supply from arteries in the neck, not the scalp. A severe scalp wound may have an accompanying skull fracture, impaled object, or spinal injury.

Care for Scalp Wounds

To care for a scalp wound:

1. Wear medical exam gloves.
2. Control bleeding by firmly applying direct pressure with a dry sterile dressing **Figure 9-1**. If the dressing becomes blood filled, do not remove it. Add another dressing on top of the first one.
3. If you suspect a skull fracture, apply pressure around the edges of the wound and over a broad area rather than on the center of the wound. Use a doughnut (ring) pad around the area.
4. Keep the head and shoulders slightly elevated to help control bleeding if you do not suspect a neck or spinal injury.
5. Seek medical care.

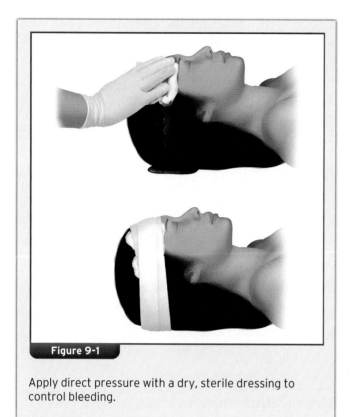

Figure 9-1

Apply direct pressure with a dry, sterile dressing to control bleeding.

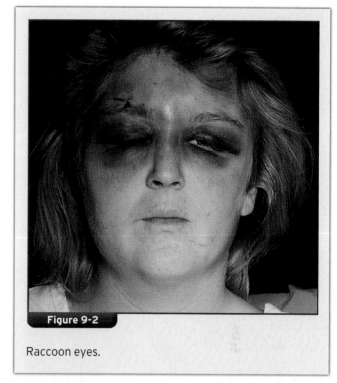

Figure 9-2

Raccoon eyes.

CAUTION

DO NOT remove an embedded object; instead stabilize it in place with bulky dressings.

DO NOT clean or irrigate a scalp wound if you suspect a skull fracture, because the fluid can carry debris and bacteria into the brain.

▶ Skull Fracture

Significant force applied to the head may cause a <u>skull fracture</u>. This occurs when part of the skull (the bones forming the head) is broken.

Recognizing a Skull Fracture

It is difficult to determine a skull fracture except by x-ray, unless the skull deformity is severe. Signs and symptoms of a skull fracture include the following:

- Pain at the point of injury.
- Deformity of the skull.
- Bleeding coming from the ears or nose.
- A clear, pink, watery fluid known as cerebrospinal fluid (CSF) leaking from an ear or the nose. A drop of CSF on a handkerchief, pillowcase, or other light-colored cloth will resemble a target, with a pink ring around a slightly blood-tinged center; this is called the *halo sign* or *ring sign*.

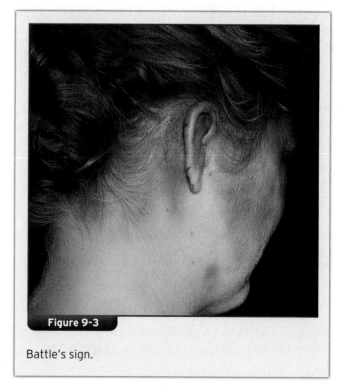

Figure 9-3

Battle's sign.

- Discoloration around the eyes ("raccoon eyes") appearing several hours after the injury **Figure 9-2** .
- Discoloration behind an ear (known as *Battle's sign*) appearing several hours after the injury **Figure 9-3** .
- Unequal sized pupils **Figure 9-4** .
- Profuse scalp bleeding if skin is broken. A scalp wound may expose the skull or brain tissue.

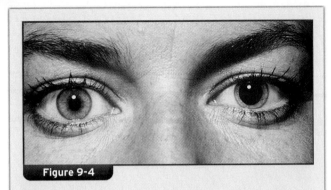

Figure 9-4

Assess pupil size if you suspect a head injury. Unequal pupil size may signal a serious problem.

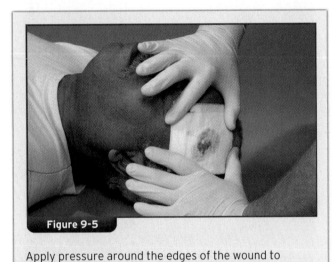

Figure 9-5

Apply pressure around the edges of the wound to control bleeding from a suspected skull fracture.

- Penetrating wound (eg, from a bullet) or impaled object.

Care for a Skull Fracture

To care for a skull fracture:
1. Monitor breathing.
2. Cover wounds with a sterile dressing.
3. Stabilize the victim's neck against movement.
4. To control bleeding, apply pressure around the edges of the wound, not directly on it **Figure 9-5**.

▶ Brain Injuries

When the head is struck with sufficient force, the brain bounces against the inside of the skull. The brain, like other body tissue, will swell from bleeding. Unlike other tissues, however, the brain is confined in the skull where there is little space for swelling. Therefore, swelling of brain tissue or accumulation of blood inside the skull compresses the brain and increases the pressure inside the skull, which interferes with brain functioning.

Recognizing a Brain Injury

The following are frequently observed signs and symptoms of a concussion, according to the American Academy of Neurology and the Brain Injury Association:
- Confused facial expression
- Slow to answer questions or follow instruction
- Easily distracted and unable to follow through with normal activities
- Walking in the wrong direction; unaware of time, date, and place
- Making disjointed or incomprehensible statements
- Stumbling, inability to walk straight line
- Distraught, crying for no apparent reason
- Asking the same question even though it has already been answered, or unable to memorize and recall three words or three objects in sequence in 5 minutes
- Coma, unresponsiveness

Care for Brain Injuries

To care for a brain injury:
1. Seek immediate medical care for all brain-injury victims.
2. Suspect a spinal injury in an unresponsive victim until proven otherwise. Stabilize the victim's head and neck against moving.
3. Monitor breathing.
4. Control bleeding by covering wounds with sterile dressings as a barrier against infection. If you suspect a skull fracture, apply pressure around the wound edges, not directly on the wound.
5. Brain-injury victims tend to vomit. Rolling the victim onto his or her side while stabilizing the neck against movement will help drain vomit and keep the airway open.

Unfortunately, there is little a first aider can do for a brain injury. The victim must be transported to the care of a neurosurgeon.

> **CAUTION**
>
> DO NOT stop the flow of blood or CSF from the ears or nose. Blocking either flow could increase pressure inside the skull.
>
> DO NOT elevate the legs—that might increase pressure on the brain.
>
> DO NOT clean an open skull injury—infection of the brain may result.

Head Injuries

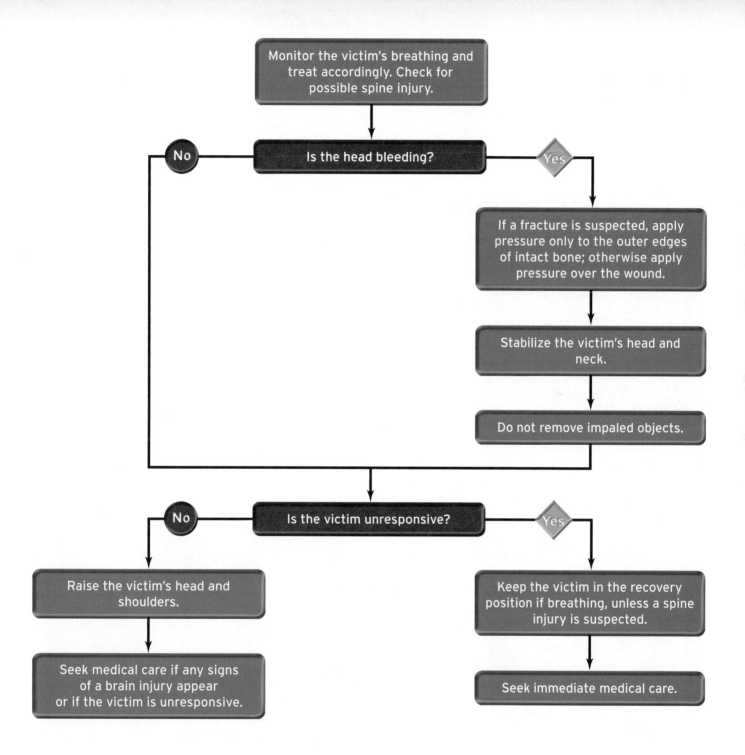

Monitor the victim's breathing and treat accordingly. Check for possible spine injury.

Is the head bleeding?

No →

Yes →

If a fracture is suspected, apply pressure only to the outer edges of intact bone; otherwise apply pressure over the wound.

Stabilize the victim's head and neck.

Do not remove impaled objects.

Is the victim unresponsive?

No →

Yes →

Raise the victim's head and shoulders.

Seek medical care if any signs of a brain injury appear or if the victim is unresponsive.

Keep the victim in the recovery position if breathing, unless a spine injury is suspected.

Seek immediate medical care.

Eye Injuries

Eye injuries can involve minor conditions such as a foreign object such as dirt in the eye. But they can also involve more severe injuries that can compromise sight if not cared for immediately. Do not assume that any eye injury is innocent. When in doubt, seek medical care immediately.

▶ Loose Foreign Objects in Eye

Loose objects in the eye are the most frequent eye injury and can be very painful. Even a small foreign object, such as a grain of sand, can produce severe irritation. Tearing is common, because it is the body's way of trying to remove the object.

Care for Loose Foreign Objects in the Eye

Try one or more of the following techniques to remove the object **Figure 9-6** :

1. Lift the upper lid over the lower lid, allowing the lashes to brush the object off the inside of the upper lid. Have the victim blink a few times and let the eye move the object out. If the object remains, keep the eye closed.
2. Try flushing the object out by rinsing the eye gently with warm water. Hold the eyelid open and tell the victim to move the eye as it is rinsed.
3. Examine the lower lid by pulling it down gently. If you can see the object, remove it with a moistened sterile gauze or clean cloth.
4. Examine the upper lid by grasping the lashes of the upper lid, placing a match stick or cotton-tipped swab across the upper lid and rolling the lid upward over the stick or swab. If you can see the object, remove it with a moistened sterile gauze or clean cloth or flush it out.

CAUTION

DO NOT allow the victim to rub the eye.

DO NOT try to remove an embedded foreign object.

DO NOT use dry cotton (cotton balls or cotton-tipped swabs) or instruments (eg, tweezers) on an eye.

▶ Penetrating Eye Injuries

Penetrating eye injuries are severe injuries that result when an object such as a needle or flying metal fragments penetrate the eye.

Care for Penetrating Eye Injuries

To care for a penetrating eye injury:

1. Seek immediate medical care. Any penetrating eye injury should be managed in the hospital.
2. Prevent the object from moving **Figure 9-7** . Stabilize a long protruding object with bulky dressings or clean cloths. You can place a protective paper cup or a piece of cardboard folded into a cone over the affected eye to prevent bumping of the object. For short objects, surround the eye without touching the object with a doughnut-shaped (ring) pad held on with a roller bandage.

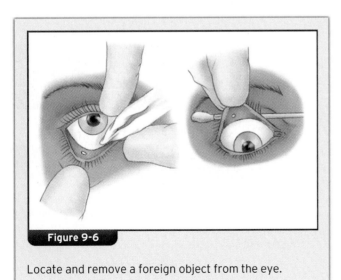

Figure 9-6

Locate and remove a foreign object from the eye.

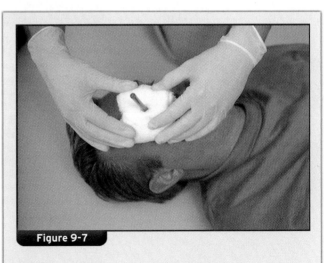

Figure 9-7

Protect a penetrating object against movement with a bulky dressing.

3. Cover the undamaged eye. Most experts suggest that the undamaged eye should be covered to prevent sympathetic eye movement (ie, the injured eye moves when the undamaged one does) and aggravating the injury. Remember that the victim is unable to see when both eyes are covered and may be anxious. Make sure you explain everything you are doing.

CAUTION

DO NOT wash out the eye with water.

DO NOT try to remove an object stuck in the eye.

DO NOT press on an injured eyeball or penetrating object.

▶ Blows to the Eye

Blows to the eye range from minor to sight threatening **Figure 9-8**.

Care for Blows to the Eye

To care for a blow to the eye:

1. Apply an ice pack immediately for about 15 minutes to reduce pain and swelling. Do not apply any pressure on the eye.
2. Seek medical care immediately if there is pain, reduced vision, or discoloration (ie, a black eye).

▶ Eye Avulsion

An <u>eye avulsion</u> occurs from a blow to the eye that knocks the eyeball from its socket.

Care for Eye Avulsion

To care for eye avulsion:

1. Cover the eye loosely with a sterile dressing that has been moistened with clean water. Do not try to push the eyeball back into the socket.
2. Protect the injured eye with a paper cup, a piece of cardboard folded into a cone, or a doughnut-shaped pad made from a roller gauze bandage or a cravat bandage.
3. Cover the undamaged eye to stop movement of the damaged eye.
4. Seek medical care immediately.

▶ Cuts of the Eye or Lid

Cuts of the eye or lid require very careful repair to restore appearance and function **Figure 9-9**.

Recognizing Cuts of the Eye or Lid

- "Cut" appearance of the cornea (clear part of the eye) or sclera (white part of the eye).
- Inner liquid of the eye may come out through the wound.
- Lid is cut.

Care for Cuts of the Eye or Lid

To care for a cut of the eye or lid:

1. If the eyeball is cut, do not apply pressure. If only the eyelid is cut, apply a sterile or clean dressing with gentle pressure.
2. Bandage both eyes lightly.
3. Seek medical care immediately.

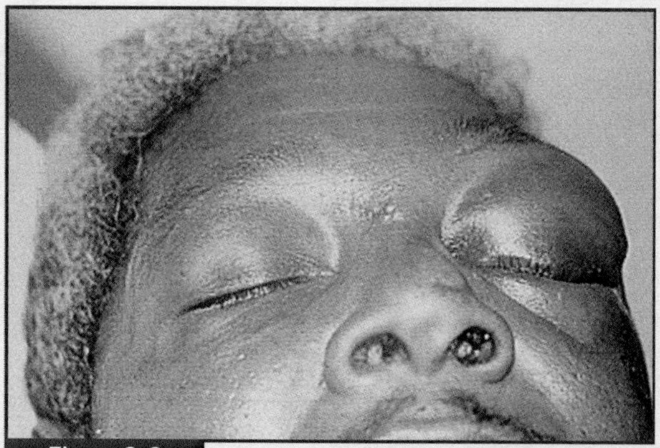

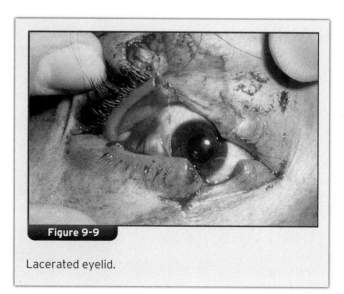

Figure 9-8

Blow to the eye.

Figure 9-9

Lacerated eyelid.

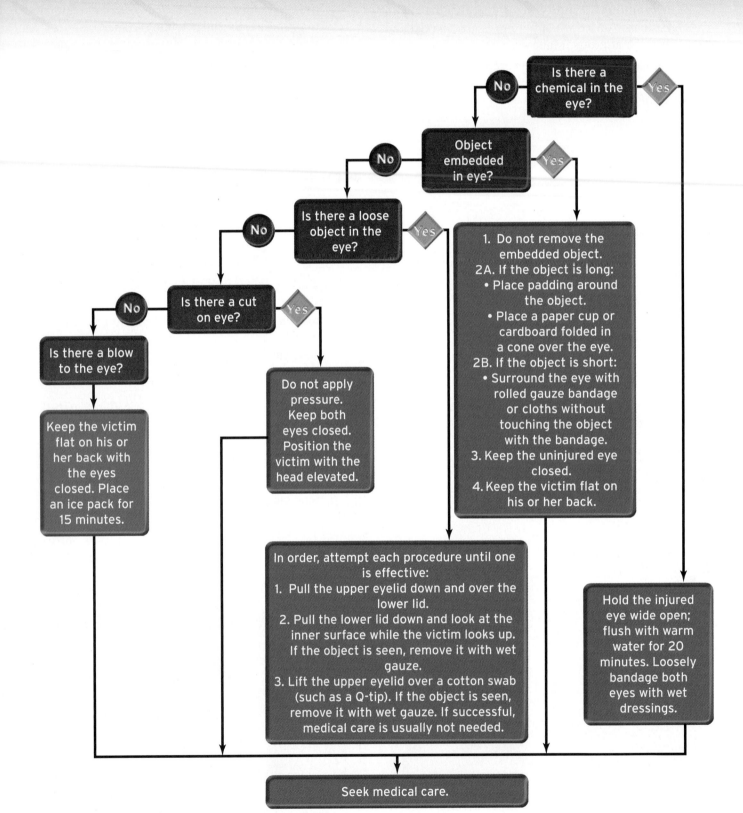

Is there a chemical in the eye?
No / Yes

Object embedded in eye?
No / Yes

Is there a loose object in the eye?
No / Yes

Is there a cut on eye?
No / Yes

Is there a blow to the eye?

Keep the victim flat on his or her back with the eyes closed. Place an ice pack for 15 minutes.

Do not apply pressure. Keep both eyes closed. Position the victim with the head elevated.

1. Do not remove the embedded object.
2A. If the object is long:
   • Place padding around the object.
   • Place a paper cup or cardboard folded in a cone over the eye.
2B. If the object is short:
   • Surround the eye with rolled gauze bandage or cloths without touching the object with the bandage.
3. Keep the uninjured eye closed.
4. Keep the victim flat on his or her back.

In order, attempt each procedure until one is effective:
1. Pull the upper eyelid down and over the lower lid.
2. Pull the lower lid down and look at the inner surface while the victim looks up. If the object is seen, remove it with wet gauze.
3. Lift the upper eyelid over a cotton swab (such as a Q-tip). If the object is seen, remove it with wet gauze. If successful, medical care is usually not needed.

Hold the injured eye wide open; flush with warm water for 20 minutes. Loosely bandage both eyes with wet dressings.

Seek medical care.

▶ Chemicals in the Eye

Chemical burns of the eyes are extremely sight threatening. First aid may determine the fate of the eye and vision. Alkalis cause greater damage than acids because they penetrate deeper and continue to burn longer. Common alkalis include drain cleaners, cleaning agents, ammonia, cement, plaster, and caustic soda. Common acids include hydrochloric acid, nitric acid, sulfuric (battery) acid, and acetic acid. Because damage can happen in 1 to 5 minutes, the chemical must be removed immediately.

Care for Chemicals in the Eye

To care for chemicals in the eye:
1. Use your fingers to keep the eye open as wide as possible.
2. Flush the eye with water immediately. If possible, use warm water. If water is not available, use any nonirritating liquid.
   a. Hold the victim's head under a faucet or pour water into the eye from any clean container for 20 minutes, continuously and gently. It is impossible to use too much water on these injuries **Figure 9-10** .
   b. Irrigate from the nose side of the eye toward the outside, to avoid flushing material into the other eye.
   c. Tell the victim to roll the eyeball as much as possible to help wash out the eye.
3. Loosely bandage both eyes with cold, wet dressings.
4. Seek immediate medical care.

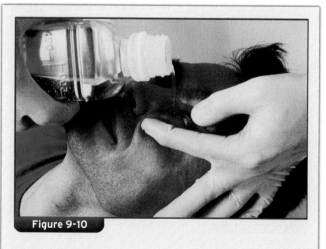

Figure 9-10

Flushing the eye to treat a chemical burn.

▶ Eye Burns From Light

Burns can result if a person looks at a source of ultraviolet light (eg, sunlight, arc welding, bright snow, tanning lamps). Severe pain begins 1 to 6 hours after exposure.

Care for Eye Burns From Light

To care for an eye burn from light:
1. Cover both eyes with cold, wet packs. Tell the victim not to rub the eyes.
2. Have the victim rest in a darkened room. Do not allow light to reach the victim's eyes.
3. Give pain medication if needed.
4. Seek medical care.

Nose Injuries

The nose often gets hit during sports activities, physical assaults, and motor vehicle crashes.

▶ Nosebleeds

Rupture of tiny blood vessels inside the nostrils by a blow to the nose, sneezing, or picking causes most nosebleeds. There are two types of nosebleeds:
- <u>Anterior (front of nose) nosebleeds</u> are the most common type (90%). Blood comes out of the nose through one nostril.
- <u>Posterior (back of nose) nosebleeds</u> involve massive bleeding backward into the mouth or down the back of the throat. A posterior nosebleed is serious and requires medical care.

Care for Nosebleeds

To care for a nosebleed:

1. Place the victim in a seated position.
2. Keep the victim's head tilted slightly forward so blood can run out the front of the nose, not down the back of the throat, which can cause choking, nausea, or vomiting.
3. Pinch (or have the victim pinch) all the soft parts of the nose together between the thumb and two fingers with steady pressure for 5 minutes **Figure 9-11**. While pinching the nostrils, push the pinched parts against the bones of the face.
4. If bleeding persists, have the victim gently sniff or blow the nose to remove any irregular clots and excess blood and to minimize sneezing. This allows new clots to form. If available, spray the nose four times on each side with a decongestant spray (Afrin™, Neo-Synephrin™), then pinch the nostrils again for 5 minutes.
5. Apply an ice pack over the nose and cheeks to help control bleeding—especially if caused by a blow to the nose.
6. Seek medical care if any of the following apply:
   - The nostril pinching and other methods do not stop the bleeding.
   - You suspect a posterior nosebleed.
   - The victim has high blood pressure or is taking anticoagulants (blood thinners) or large doses of aspirin.
   - Bleeding happens after a blow to the nose, and you suspect a broken nose.

▶ Broken Nose

A blow to the nose can break the nose.

Recognizing a Broken Nose

To recognize a broken nose, look for:
- Pain, swelling, and a possible crooked appearance.
- Bleeding and difficulty breathing through the nostrils.
- Black eyes appearing 1 to 2 days after the injury.

Care for a Broken Nose

To care for a broken nose:

1. Treat a nosebleed as described above.
2. Apply an ice pack to the nose for 15 minutes. Do not try to straighten a crooked nose.
3. Seek medical care.

Mouth Injuries

Because mouth emergencies generally cause considerable pain and anxiety, managing them promptly can provide great relief to the victim.

▶ Knocked-Out Tooth

A knocked-out tooth is a common dental emergency **Figure 9-12**. More than 90% of the 2 million teeth knocked out each year in the United States could be saved with proper treatment.

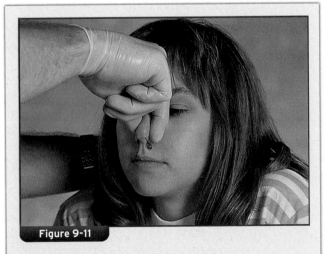

Figure 9-11

Control bleeding from the nose by pinching the nostrils together.

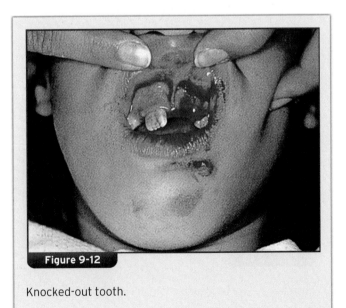

Figure 9-12

Knocked-out tooth.

Nosebleeds

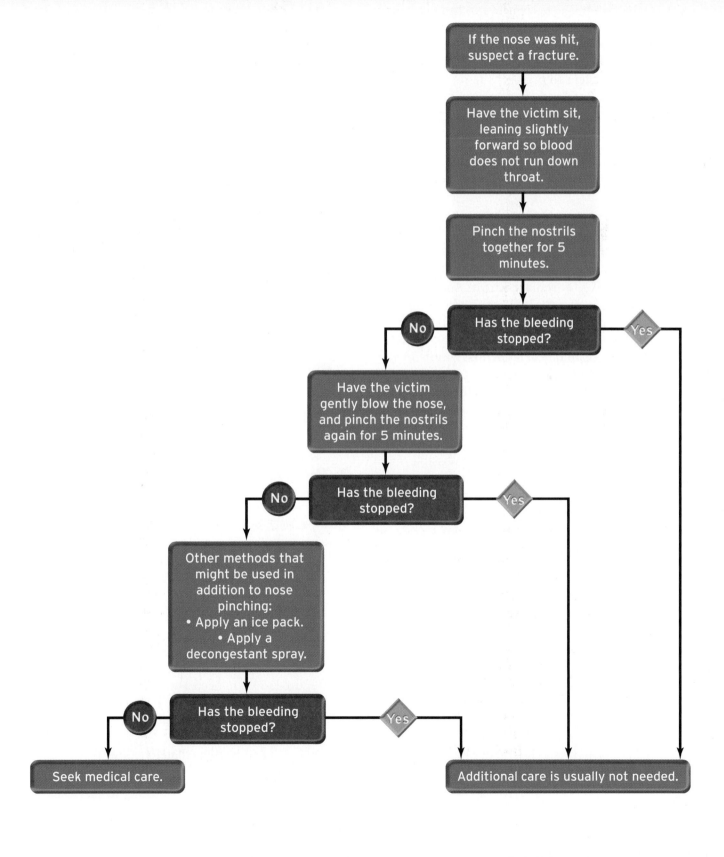

If the nose was hit, suspect a fracture.

Have the victim sit, leaning slightly forward so blood does not run down throat.

Pinch the nostrils together for 5 minutes.

No ← Has the bleeding stopped? → **Yes**

Have the victim gently blow the nose, and pinch the nostrils again for 5 minutes.

No ← Has the bleeding stopped? → **Yes**

Other methods that might be used in addition to nose pinching:
• Apply an ice pack.
• Apply a decongestant spray.

No ← Has the bleeding stopped? → **Yes**

Seek medical care.

Additional care is usually not needed.

Care for a Knocked-Out Tooth

Emergency care for knocked-out teeth has changed dramatically in recent years. The first question you want to ask in this situation is, "Where is the tooth?" Time is crucial for successful reimplantation. After a tooth is knocked out, ligament fiber fragments remain attached to the tooth and to the bone in the socket. However, the ligament fibers begin to die soon after the injury. Therefore, it is important to prevent the tooth from drying. Moisture alone is not sufficient to preserve the tooth's ligament fibers. Steps must be taken both to prevent the tooth from becoming dehydrated and to protect the ligament fibers from damage.

To care for a knocked-out tooth:

1. Have the victim rinse his or her mouth and put a rolled gauze pad in the socket to control bleeding.
2. Find the tooth and handle it by the crown, not the root, to minimize damage to the ligament fibers.
3. The best place for a knocked-out tooth is its socket. A tooth often can be successfully reimplanted if it is replaced in its socket within 30 minutes after the injury; the odds of successful reimplantation decrease about 1% for every minute the tooth is absent from the socket. If the victim cannot reach a dentist within 30 minutes, try to place the tooth into the socket, using adjacent teeth as a guide. If the tooth is dirty, gently rinse with milk or the victim's saliva. Do not rinse with water. Apply pressure on the tooth so the top is even with the adjacent teeth. Immediate reinsertion is not always possible, however. The victim may be reluctant to put the knocked-out tooth back into its socket, especially if it has fallen on the ground and is covered with debris. Or the tooth may repeatedly fall out, putting the victim at risk of inhaling or swallowing it. In victims with multiple trauma, the presence of more serious injuries may prevent reinsertion. When immediate reinsertion is not possible, the tooth should be transported in cool milk. Some experts recommend that the tooth be placed in the victim's mouth to keep it moist until dental treatment is available. This method, although convenient, presents the risk that the tooth could be swallowed, especially by children.
4. Take the victim and the tooth to a dentist immediately even if it has been reinserted.

> ## CAUTION
>
> DO NOT place a knocked-out tooth in skim milk, powdered milk, or milk by-products such as yogurt.
>
> DO NOT rinse a knocked-out tooth unless you are reinserting it in the socket.
>
> DO NOT scrub a knocked-out tooth or remove any attached tissue fragments found on the tooth's roots.
>
> DO NOT remove a partially extracted tooth. Push it back into place and seek a dentist so the loose tooth can be stabilized.

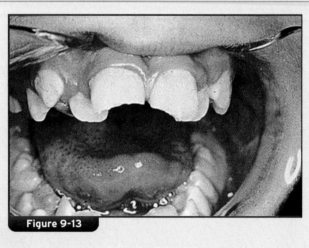

Figure 9-13

Broken teeth.

▶ Broken Tooth

The front teeth are frequently broken by falls or direct blows **Figure 9-13** . Such damage can occur in motor-vehicle crashes, sports, and violent acts.

Care for a Broken Tooth

To care for a broken tooth:

1. Gently clean dirt and blood from the injured area with a sterile gauze pad or a clean cloth and warm water.
2. Apply an ice pack to the face in the area of the injured tooth to decrease swelling.
3. If you suspect a jaw fracture, stabilize the jaw by wrapping a bandage under the chin and over the top of the head.
4. Seek a dentist immediately.

Dental Injuries

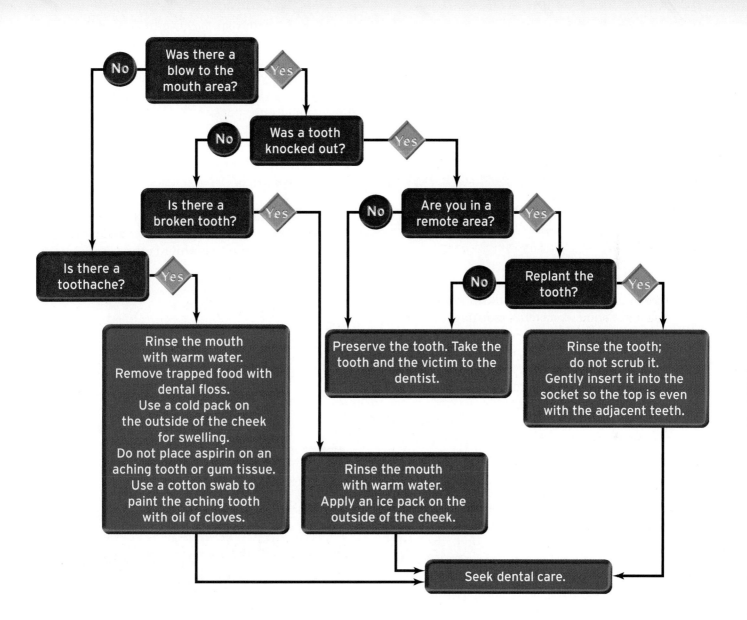

Was there a blow to the mouth area?
- No
- Yes

Was a tooth knocked out?
- No
- Yes

Is there a broken tooth?
- Yes

Are you in a remote area?
- No
- Yes

Is there a toothache?
- Yes

Replant the tooth?
- No
- Yes

Rinse the mouth with warm water. Remove trapped food with dental floss. Use a cold pack on the outside of the cheek for swelling. Do not place aspirin on an aching tooth or gum tissue. Use a cotton swab to paint the aching tooth with oil of cloves.

Preserve the tooth. Take the tooth and the victim to the dentist.

Rinse the tooth; do not scrub it. Gently insert it into the socket so the top is even with the adjacent teeth.

Rinse the mouth with warm water. Apply an ice pack on the outside of the cheek.

Seek dental care.

▶ Toothache

The tooth will be sensitive to heat and cold. Identify the diseased tooth by tapping the area with a spoon handle or similar object. A diseased tooth will hurt.

Care for Toothaches

To care for toothaches:
1. Rinse the mouth with warm water to clean it out.
2. Use dental floss to remove any food that might be trapped between the teeth.
3. Give the victim pain medication such as ibuprofen.
4. Seek a dentist immediately.

Spinal Injuries

Head injuries serve as a clue to possible spinal injuries because the head may have been moved suddenly in one or more directions, damaging the spine.

Recognizing Spinal Injuries

The signs of a spinal injury include the following:
- Pain in the spine, sometimes radiating to the arms or legs
- Numbness, tingling, weakness, or burning sensation in the arms or legs
- Loss of bowel or bladder control
- Paralysis of the arms or legs
- Deformity (odd-looking angle of the victim's head and neck)

If the victim is responsive, ask these questions and follow these steps:
- *Is there pain?* Neck (cervical spine) injuries radiate pain to the arms; upper-back (thoracic spine) injuries radiate pain around the ribs; lower-back injuries usually radiate pain down the legs. Often, the victim describes the pain as "electric." See **Skill Drill 9-1**.

For each hand:
- *Can you wiggle your fingers?* Moving the fingers is a sign that nerve pathways are intact (**Step ❶**).
- *Can you feel this pressure on your fingers?* Pinch several tips of the victim's fingers to check for spinal injury (**Step ❷**).
- *Can you squeeze my hand?* Ask the victim to grip your hand. A strong grip indicates that an upper spinal cord injury is unlikely (**Step ❸**).

For each foot:
- *Can you wiggle your toes?* Moving the toes is a sign that nerve pathways are intact (**Step ❹**).
- *Can you feel pressure on your toes?* Pinch several tips of the victim's toes to check for spinal injury (**Step ❺**).
- *Can you push your foot against my hand?* Ask the victim to press a foot against your hand. If the victim cannot perform this movement or the movement is extremely weak against your hand, the victim may have a spinal injury (**Step ❻**).

If the victim is unresponsive, do the following:
- Look for cuts, bruises, and deformities.
- Test responses by pinching the victim's hand (either palm or back of the hand) and bare foot (sole or top of the foot). No reaction could mean spinal damage.
- Ask bystanders what happened. If you still are not sure about a possible spinal injury, assume the victim has one until it is proved otherwise.

Care for a Spinal Injury

To care for a spinal injury:
1. Stabilize the victim against any movement **Figure 9-14**.
2. Monitor breathing.
3. Call 9-1-1.

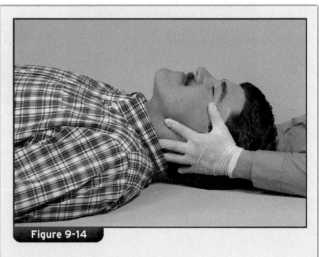

Figure 9-14

Prevent movement of the head and neck.

skill drill

9-1 Checking for Spinal Injuries in a Responsive Victim

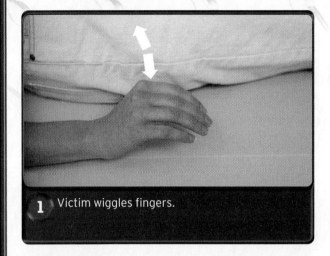

1 Victim wiggles fingers.

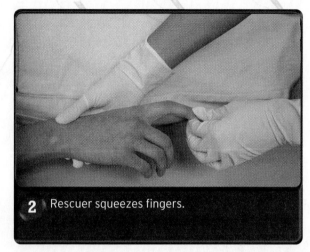

2 Rescuer squeezes fingers.

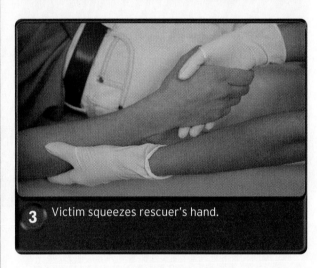

3 Victim squeezes rescuer's hand.

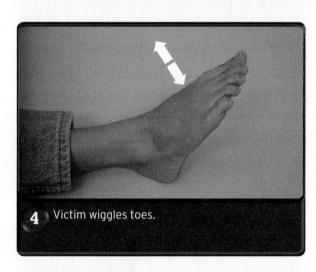

4 Victim wiggles toes.

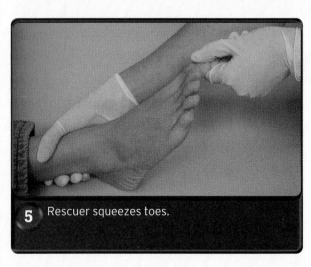

5 Rescuer squeezes toes.

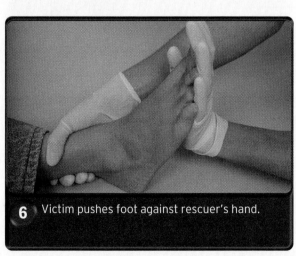

6 Victim pushes foot against rescuer's hand.

Spinal Injuries

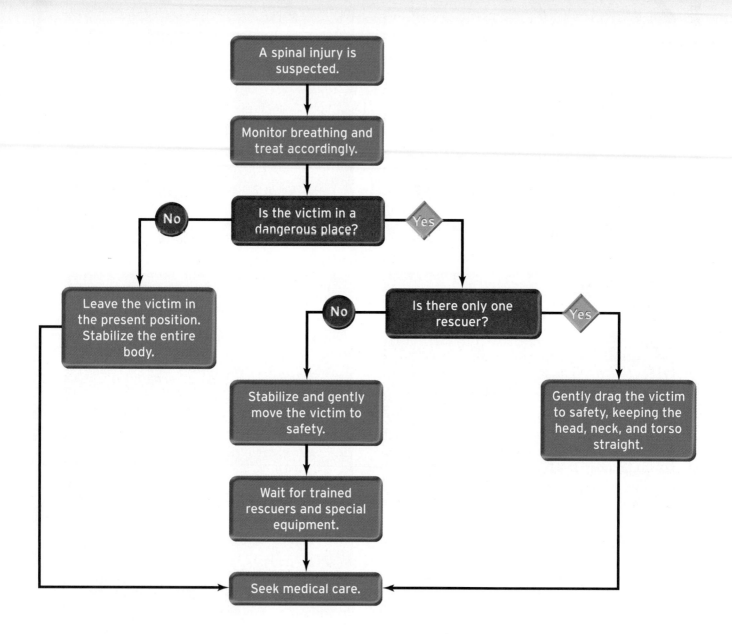

▶ Head Injuries

What to Look For	**What to Do**
Scalp wound	1. Apply a sterile or clean dressing and direct pressure to control bleeding. 2. Keep head and shoulders raised. 3. Seek medical care.
Skull fracture • Pain at point of injury • Deformity of the skull • Clear or bloody fluid draining from ears or nose • Bruising under eyes or behind an ear • Changes in pupils • Heavy scalp bleeding • Penetrating wound	1. Monitor breathing and provide care if needed. 2. Control bleeding by applying pressure around the edges of wound. 3. Stabilize the victim's head and neck against movement. 4. Seek medical care.
Brain injury (concussion) • Befuddled facial expression (vacant stare) • Slowness in answering questions • Unawareness of where they are or day of week • Slurred speech • Stumbling, inability to walk a straight line • Crying for no apparent reason • Inability to recite months of year in reverse order • Unresponsiveness • Headache, dizziness, and nausea	1. Monitor breathing and provide care if needed. 2. Stabilize the victim's head and neck against movement. 3. Control any scalp bleeding. 4. Seek medical care.

▶ Eye Injuries

What to Look For	**What to Do**
Loose foreign object in eye	1. Look for object underneath both lids. 2. If seen, remove with wet gauze.
Penetrating eye injury	1. If object is still in eye, protect eye and stabilize long objects. 2. Call 9-1-1.
Blow to the eye	1. Apply an ice or cold pack. DO NOT place ice or cold pack on eyeball. 2. Seek medical care if vision is affected.
Eye avulsion • Eyeball knocked out of its socket	1. Cover eye loosely with wet dressing. 2. DO NOT try to put eye back into socket. 3. Call 9-1-1.
Cuts of eye or lid	1. If eyeball is cut, DO NOT apply pressure. 2. If only eyelid is cut, apply dressing with gentle pressure. 3. Call 9-1-1.
Chemicals in eye	1. Flush with warm water for 20 minutes and loosely bandage with wet dressings. 2. Seek medical care.
Eye burns from light	1. Cover eyes with cold, wet dressings. 2. Seek medical care.

▶ Nose Injuries

What to Look For	What to Do

Nosebleeds	1. Keep victim sitting up with head level or tilted forward slightly.
	2. Pinch soft parts of nose for 5 to 10 minutes.
	3. Seek medical care if:
	   • Bleeding does not stop
	   • Blood is going down throat
	   • Bleeding is associated with a broken nose

Broken nose • Pain, swelling, and possibly crooked nose • Bleeding and breathing difficulty through nostrils • Black eyes appearing 1 to 2 days after injury	1. Care for nosebleed. 2. Apply an ice or cold pack for 15 minutes. 3. Seek medical care.

▶ Mouth Injuries

What to Look For	What to Do
Bitten lip or tongue	1. Apply direct pressure. 2. Apply an ice or cold pack.
Knocked-out tooth	1. Control bleeding (place rolled gauze in socket). 2. Find tooth and preserve it in milk or the victim's saliva. Handle the tooth by the crown, not the root. 3. See dentist as soon as possible.
Toothache	1. Rinse mouth and use dental floss to removed trapped food. 2. Give pain medication. 3. Seek dental care.

▶ Spinal Injuries

What to Look For	What to Do
• Inability to move arms and/or legs • Numbness, tingling, weakness, or burning feeling in arms and/or legs • Deformity (head and neck at an odd angle) • Neck or back pain	1. Stabilize the head and neck against movement. 2. If unresponsive, open the victim's airway and check breathing. 3. Call 9-1-1.

▶ Ready for Review

- Any head injury is potentially serious and may be life threatening.
- Scalp wounds bleed profusely because the scalp has a rich supply of blood and the blood vessels do not constrict.
- A skull fracture is a break or crack in the cranium.
- Penetrating eye injuries can potentially cause the loss of vision.
- Loose objects in the eye are the most frequent eye injury.
- Chemicals in the eye require irrigation with water for 20 minutes.
- Burns to the eye can result if a person looks at a source of ultraviolet light.
- Most nosebleeds do not require medical care and can be control by pinching the nose for 5 minutes.
- A knocked-out tooth should be replaced within 30 minutes.
- Dental decay is the main cause of toothaches.
- Spinal injured victims are best handled by those with training and the correct equipment.

▶ Vital Vocabulary

anterior (front of nose) nosebleed The most common type (90%) of nosebleed. Blood comes out of the nose through one nostril.

eye avulsion Occurs from a blow to the eye that knocks the eyeball from its socket.

posterior (back of nose) nosebleed Involves massive bleeding backward into the mouth or down the back of the throat. A posterior nosebleed is serious and requires medical care.

skull fracture This occurs when part of the skull (the bones forming the head) is broken.

▶ Assessment in Action

You see a middle-aged man walking down the street; suddenly, he is struck by a piece of wood that has fallen 50 feet from a construction site above. The victim collapses and remains on the ground. He is slow to answer questions and cannot remember where he is or the day of the week. He says he feels lightheaded and nauseated. You see a lot of blood coming from a wound on his head.
Directions: Circle *Yes* if you agree with the statement and *No* if you disagree.

Yes   No   1. The victim should be checked for a possible spinal injury.

Yes   No   2. To treat for shock, this victim should be placed flat on his back with his legs elevated.

Yes   No   3. You do not suspect a concussion because the victim is still alert.

Yes   No   4. Stabilize the head and neck against movement.

Answers: 1. Yes; 2. No; 3. No; 4. Yes

▶ Check Your Knowledge

Directions: Circle *Yes* if you agree with the statement and *No* if you disagree.

Yes   No   1. To control bleeding, press around the edges of a suspected skull fracture and not directly on the wound.

Yes   No   2. Do NOT remove impaled (embedded) objects.

Yes   No   3. Victims with head injuries should be checked for a possible spinal injury.

Yes   No   4. After a blow to an eye, apply a cold pack for about 15 minutes.

Yes   No   5. Tears are sufficient to flush a chemical from the eye.

Yes   No   6. Use a clean, damp cloth to remove an object from the eyelid's surface.

Yes   No   7. Preserve a knocked-out tooth in mouthwash or rubbing alcohol.

Yes   No   8. Scrub a knocked-out tooth before taking the victim to a dentist.

Yes   No   9. Do NOT move a victim with a suspected spinal injury.

Yes   No   10. Inability to move fingers and/or feet may indicate a spinal injury.

Answers: 1. Yes; 2. Yes; 3. Yes; 4. Yes; 5. No; 6. Yes; 7. No; 8. No; 9. Yes; 10. Yes

Chest, Abdominal, and Pelvic Injuries

▶ Chest Injuries

Chest injuries can be closed or open. In a <u>closed chest injury</u>, the victim's skin is not broken. This type of injury is usually caused by blunt trauma. In an <u>open chest injury</u>, the skin has been broken and the chest wall is penetrated by an object such as a knife or bullet. All chest injury victims should be checked and rechecked for breathing. A responsive chest injury victim should usually sit up or be placed with the injured side down. This position protects the uninjured side from blood inside the chest cavity and allows the uninjured side to expand.

Recognizing Rib Fractures

Rib fractures are a closed chest injury. The most common type of rib fracture is ribs fractured by a blow or a fall. A <u>flail chest</u> results when several ribs in the same area are broken in more than one place. Rib fractures usually occur along the side of the chest.

The signs of a rib fracture include:

- Sharp pain when the victim breathes, coughs, or moves and pain at the injured site
- Shallow breathing because of the pain
- Victim holds the injured area, trying to reduce the pain (this is known as *guarding*)
- Pain produced when gently squeezing the chest during the physical exam
- Coughing up blood or pink frothy fluid due to a punctured lung.

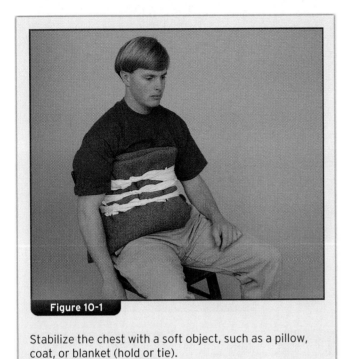

Figure 10-1

Stabilize the chest with a soft object, such as a pillow, coat, or blanket (hold or tie).

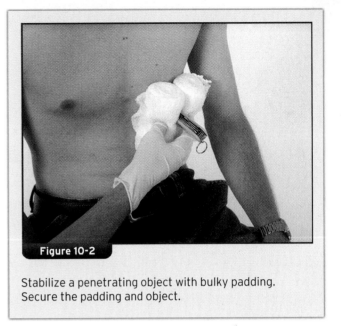

Figure 10-2

Stabilize a penetrating object with bulky padding. Secure the padding and object.

Care for Rib Fractures

To care for a rib fracture:

1. Help the victim find a comfortable resting position.
2. Stabilize the ribs by having the victim hold a pillow or other similar soft object against the injured area **Figure 10-1** . Or, use bandages to hold the pillow in place or tie an arm over the injured area. Do not apply tight bandages around the chest, because they restrict breathing.
3. Some victims find comfort by lying on the injured side.
4. Seek medical care.

Recognizing an Embedded (Impaled) Object

An impaled object is usually easily recognized. However, in some cases the object may be below the skin surface and is difficult to see.

Care for an Embedded (Impaled) Object

To care for an embedded (impaled) object:

1. Stabilize the object in place with bulky dressings **Figure 10-2** . *Do not try to remove an impaled object*—bleeding and air in the chest cavity can result.
2. Seek medical care.

Recognizing a Sucking Chest Wound

A <u>sucking chest wound</u> results when a chest wound allows air to pass into and out of the chest cavity with each breath. The signs of a sucking chest wound include:

- Blood bubbling out of a chest wound
- The sound of air being sucked into and out of the chest wound

Care for a Sucking Chest Wound

To care for a sucking chest wound:

1. Have the victim take a breath and let it out, then seal the wound with anything available to stop air from entering the chest cavity. Plastic wrap or a plastic bag works well. Tape it in place but leave one side untaped **Figure 10-3** . This creates a flutter valve to prevent air from being trapped in the chest cavity. If plastic wrap is not available, you can use your gloved hand.
2. If the victim has trouble breathing or seems to be getting worse, remove the plastic cover (or your hand) to let air escape, then reapply.
3. Call 9-1-1.

▶ Abdominal Injuries

Abdominal injuries are either open or closed. <u>Closed abdominal injuries</u> occur as the result of a direct blow from a blunt object. <u>Open abdominal injuries</u> include penetrating wounds, embedded (impaled) objects, and protruding organs.

Chest Injuries

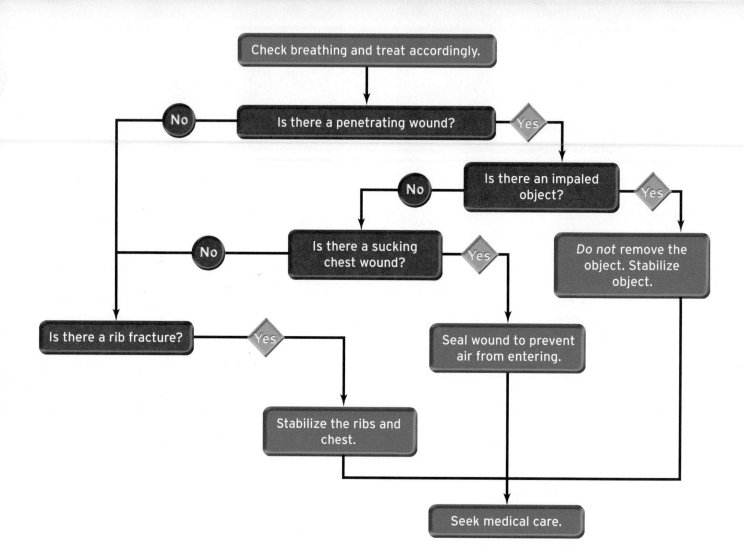

Check breathing and treat accordingly.

Is there a penetrating wound?   No / Yes

Is there an impaled object?   No / Yes

Is there a sucking chest wound?   No / Yes

Do not remove the object. Stabilize object.

Is there a rib fracture?   Yes

Seal wound to prevent air from entering.

Stabilize the ribs and chest.

Seek medical care.

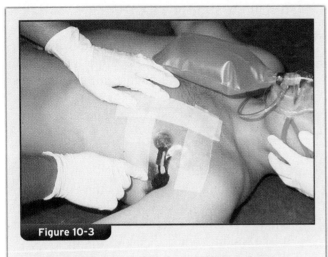

Figure 10-3

For a sucking chest wound, tape three sides of the plastic in place.

Recognizing a Closed Abdominal Injury

Examine the abdomen by gently pressing different areas of the abdomen with your fingertips. Observe for pain, tenderness, muscle tightness, or rigidity. A normal abdomen is soft and not tender when pressed. Signs of a closed abdominal injury include:

- Bruises or other marks
- Pain, tenderness, muscle tightness or rigidity

Care for a Closed Abdominal Injury

To care for a closed abdominal injury:

1. Place the victim in a comfortable position with the legs pulled up toward the abdomen.
2. Do not give the victim any food or drink. Expect the victim to vomit.
3. If you are hours from medical care, allow the victim to suck on a clean cloth soaked in water to relieve a dry mouth.
4. Seek medical care.

Recognizing a Penetrating Wound

To recognize a penetrating wound:

- Look for an impaled object. An impaled object is usually easily recognized. However, in some cases the object may be below the skin surface and be difficult to see.
- Bleeding may be present.

Care for a Penetrating Wound

It is difficult to know whether a penetrating injury has damaged internal organs. To care for a penetrating wound:

1. If the penetrating object is still in place, stabilize the object and control bleeding by using bulky dressings around it. *Do not try to remove the object.*
2. Seek medical care.

Recognizing a Protruding Organ

A <u>protruding organ injury</u> refers to severe injury to the abdomen in which the internal organs escape or protrude from the wound.

Care for a Protruding Organ

To care for a protruding organ:

1. Place the victim with head and shoulders slightly raised, and the knees bent and the legs pulled up toward the abdomen.
2. Cover protruding organs with a moist sterile dressing, clean cloth, or clean plastic wrap **Figure 10-4 A, B**. Keep the dressing moist and place a towel lightly over the dressing to help maintain warmth.
3. Call 9-1-1.

CAUTION

DO NOT try to reinsert protruding organs into the abdomen—you could introduce infection or damage the intestines.

DO NOT cover the organs tightly.

DO NOT cover the organs with any material that clings or disintegrates when wet.

DO NOT give the victim anything to eat or drink.

▶ Pelvic Injuries

Injuries to the pelvis are usually caused by a motor-vehicle crash or a fall. Pelvic fractures can be life-threatening because of the large amount of blood that could be lost due to internal bleeding.

Recognizing Pelvic Fractures

The signs of a pelvic injury include:

- Pain in the hip, groin, or back that increases with movement.

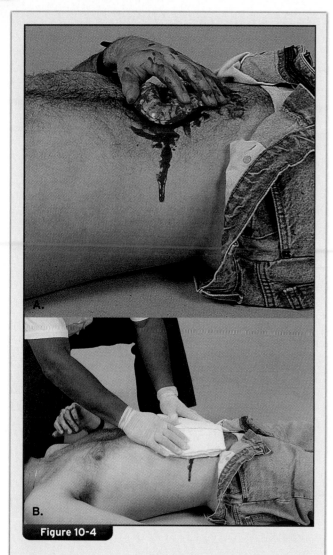

A.

B.

Figure 10-4

Bandaging an open abdominal wound. **A.** Open abdominal wounds are serious injuries. **B.** Cover organs with a moist, sterile or clean dressing.

- Inability to stand or walk.
- Signs of shock.
- Gently press the sides of the pelvis downward and squeeze them inward at the upper points of the hips. If this pressing and squeezing produces pain, suspect a broken pelvis. If the victim is already complaining about pain, do not press or squeeze.

Care for Pelvic Fractures

To care for a pelvic injury:

1. Place padding between the victim's thighs, then tie the victim's knees and ankles together. If the victim is on his or her back, bend the knees and place padding under them for support.
2. Keep the victim on a firm surface.
3. Seek medical care.

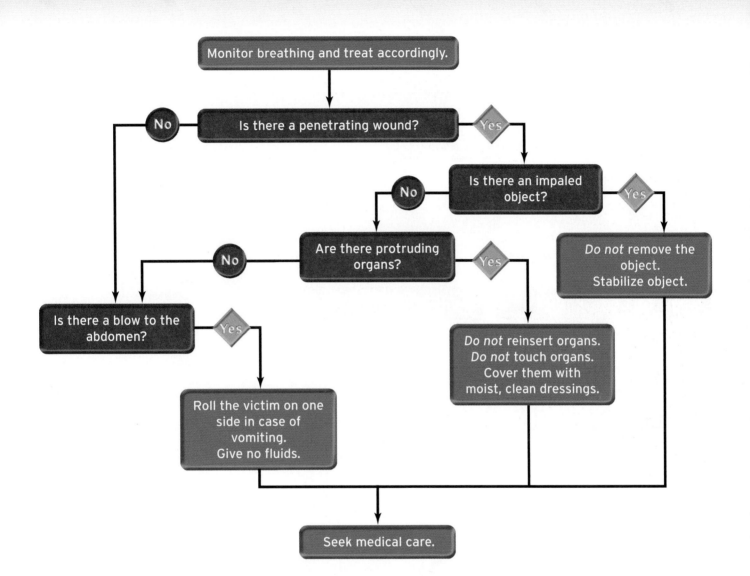

Monitor breathing and treat accordingly.

Is there a penetrating wound?

No

Yes

Is there an impaled object?

No

Yes

Do *not* remove the object.
Stabilize object.

Are there protruding organs?

No

Yes

Do *not* reinsert organs.
Do *not* touch organs.
Cover them with moist, clean dressings.

Is there a blow to the abdomen?

Yes

Roll the victim on one side in case of vomiting.
Give no fluids.

Seek medical care.

▶ Chest Injuries

What to Look For	What to Do

Rib fractures
- Sharp pain with deep breaths, coughing, or moving
- Shallow breathing
- Holding of injured area to reduce pain
- Tenderness directly on the ribs

1. Place victim in comfortable position.
2. Support ribs with a pillow, blanket, or coat (either holding or tying with bandages).
3. Seek medical care.

Embedded (impaled) object
- Object remains in wound

1. DO NOT remove object from wound.
2. Use bulky dressings or cloths to stabilize the object.
3. Call 9-1-1.

Sucking chest wound
- Blood bubbling out of wound
- Sound of air being sucked in and out of wound

1. Seal wound to stop air from entering chest; tape three sides of plastic or use gloved hand.
2. Remove cover to let air escape if victim worsens or has trouble breathing.
3. Call 9-1-1.

▶ Abdominal Injuries

What to Look For	What to Do

Blow to abdomen (closed)
- Bruise or other marks
- Muscle tightness and rigidity felt while gently pushing on abdomen

1. Place victim in comfortable position with legs pulled up toward the abdomen.
2. Care for shock.
3. Seek medical care.

Protruding organs (open)
- Internal organs escaping from abdominal wound

1. Place victim in a comfortable position with the legs pulled up toward the abdomen.
2. DO NOT reinsert organs into the abdomen.
3. Cover organs with a moist, sterile or clean dressing.
4. Care for shock.
5. Call 9-1-1.

▶ Pelvic Injuries

What to Look For	What to Do

Pelvic fractures
- Pain in hip, groin, or back that increases with movement
- Inability to walk or stand
- Signs of shock

1. Keep victim still.
2. Care for shock.
3. Call 9-1-1.

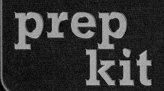

prep kit

▶ Ready for Review

- Chest injuries fall into two categories: open or closed.
- Closed chest injuries include rib fractures and flail chest.
- In an open chest injury, the skin is broken and the chest wall is penetrated by an object such as a knife or bullet.
- Abdominal injuries are either open or closed and can involve internal organs.
- Closed abdominal injuries occur when the internal abdominal tissues and/or organs are damaged but the skin is unbroken.
- Open abdominal injuries are those in which the skin has been broken. Never try to replace protruding organs.
- Pelvic fractures can involve a large amount of bleeding.

▶ Vital Vocabulary

<u>closed abdominal injuries</u> Injuries to the abdomen that occur as a result of a direct blow from a blunt object and there is no break in the skin.

<u>closed chest injury</u> An injury to the chest in which the skin is not broken; usually due to blunt trauma.

<u>flail chest</u> A condition that occurs when several ribs in the same area are broken in more than one place.

<u>open abdominal injuries</u> Injuries to the abdomen that include penetrating wounds and protruding organs.

<u>open chest injury</u> An injury to the chest in which the chest wall itself is penetrated, either by a fractured rib or, more frequently, by an external object such as a bullet or knife.

<u>protruding organ injury</u> A severe injury to the abdomen in which the internal organs escape or protrude from the wound.

<u>sucking chest wound</u> A chest wound that allows air to pass into and out of the chest cavity with each breath.

▶ Assessment in Action

A 30-year-old man fell while carrying a heavy box down stairs, missed the last two steps and landed on a garbage can. He tells you that his "stomach" landed on the garbage can and that it is hurting. While checking his abdomen, you notice a bruise marking where he hit the can.

Directions: Circle *Yes* if you agree with the statement and *No* if you disagree.

Yes   No   **1.** The victim's injury is a closed abdominal injury.

Yes   No   **2.** Your exam will include gently pressing on the abdomen.

Yes   No   **3.** Give the victim something to drink.

Yes   No   **4.** Because there is no bleeding, medical care is not needed.

Answers: 1. Yes; 2. Yes; 3. No; 4. No

▶ Check Your Knowledge

Directions: Circle *Yes* if you agree with the statement and *No* if you disagree.

Yes   No   **1.** Stabilize a broken rib by strapping (taping) a victim's chest as tightly as possible.

Yes   No   **2.** Stabilize an impaled (embedded) object in the chest with bulky padding to prevent it from moving.

Yes   No   **3.** Cover a sucking chest wound with plastic wrap.

Yes   No   **4.** Gently push protruding organs back through the abdominal wound.

Yes   No   **5.** The dressing covering exposed intestines should be kept dry.

Yes   No   **6.** Remove any penetrating object from the abdomen.

Yes   No   **7.** For a blow to the abdomen with suspected internal injuries, pull the knees up toward the abdomen.

Yes   No   **8.** Keep the victim with a suspected pelvic fracture on a firm surface.

Yes   No   **9.** Sharp pain while breathing after being hit in the chest can be a sign of a rib fracture.

Yes   No   **10.** A broken pelvis can involve a large amount of internal bleeding.

Answers: 1. No; 2. Yes; 3. Yes; 4. No; 5. No; 6. No; 7. Yes; 8. Yes; 9. Yes; 10. Yes

Bone, Joint, and Muscle Injuries

▶ Bone Injuries

The terms <u>fracture</u> and *broken bone* have the same meaning: a break or crack in a bone. There are two categories of fractures **Figure 11-1** :

- <u>Closed fracture</u>. The skin is intact, and no wound exists anywhere near the fracture site **Figure 11-2** .
- <u>Open fracture</u>. The skin over the fracture has been damaged or broken **Figure 11-3** . The wound may result from bone protruding through the skin or by a direct blow that cuts the skin at the time of the fracture. The bone may not always be visible in the wound.

In addition to the broken bones themselves, there can be injuries to the vital structures next to them, such as internal organs, blood vessels, and nerves.

Recognizing Bone Injuries

It may be difficult to tell if a bone is fractured. When in doubt, treat the injury as a fracture. Use the mnemonic DOTS (*deformity, open wound, tenderness, swelling*) to guide your physical exam.

- *Deformity* may not be obvious. Compare the injured part with the uninjured part on the other side.
- *Open wound* may indicate an underlying fracture.
- *Tenderness* and pain commonly are found only at the injury site. Usually, the victim will be able to point to the site of the pain. A useful procedure

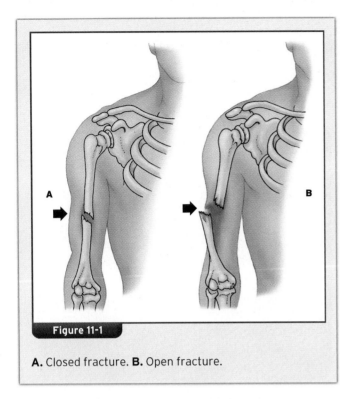

Figure 11-1

A. Closed fracture. **B.** Open fracture.

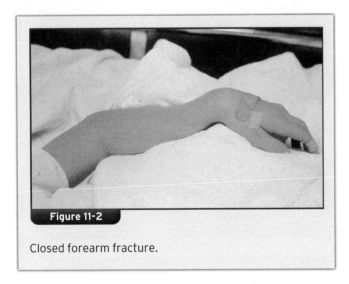

Figure 11-2

Closed forearm fracture.

for detecting a fracture is to gently feel along the bone; a victim's complaint about pain or tenderness serves as a reliable sign of a fracture.

- *Swelling* caused by bleeding happens rapidly after a fracture.

Additional signs and symptoms include:

- Loss of use may or may not occur. The victim may refuse to use the injured part if motion produces pain. This is called *guarding*. Sometimes, however, the victim is able to move a fractured limb with little or no pain.

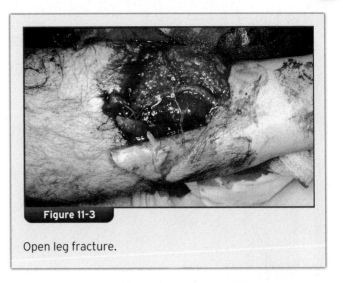

Figure 11-3

Open leg fracture.

- A grating sensation can be felt and sometimes even heard when the ends of the broken bone rub together. Do not move the injured limb in an attempt to detect it.
- The history of the injury can lead you to suspect a fracture whenever a serious accident has happened. The victim may have heard or felt the bone snap.

Care for Bone Injuries

To care for a bone injury:

1. Determine what happened and the location of the injury.
2. Gently remove clothing covering the injured area. Cut clothing at the seams if necessary.
3. Examine the area by looking and feeling for DOTS:
   - Look at the injury site. Swelling and black-and-blue marks, which indicate that blood is escaping into the tissues, may come from either the bone end or associated muscular and blood vessel damage. Shortening or severe deformity (angulation) between the joints, deformity around the joints, shortening of the extremity, and rotation of the extremity when compared with the opposite extremity indicate a bone injury. Lacerations or even small puncture wounds near the site of a bone fracture are considered open fractures.
   - Feel the injured area. If a fracture is not obvious, gently press, touch, or feel along the length of the bone for deformities, tenderness, and swelling.
4. Check blood flow and nerves. Use the mnemonic CSM (*circulation, sensation, movement*) as a way of remembering what to do (**Skill Drill 11-1**):
   - *Circulation.* Feel for the radial pulse (located on the thumb side of the wrist) for an arm injury (**Step 1a**) and the posterior tibial pulse (located

skill drill

11-1 Checking CSM in an Extremity

Upper Extremity	Lower Extremity

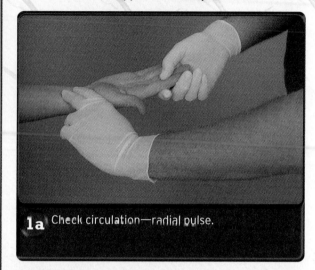

1a Check circulation—radial pulse.

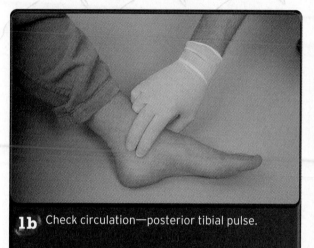

1b Check circulation—posterior tibial pulse.

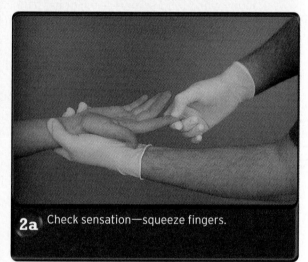

2a Check sensation—squeeze fingers.

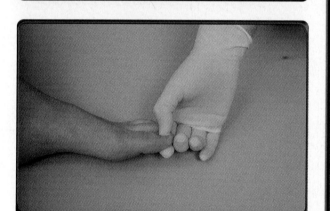

2b Check sensation—squeeze toes.

3a Check movement—wiggle fingers.

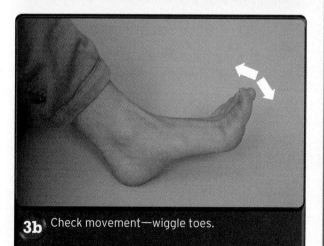

3b Check movement—wiggle toes.

between the inside ankle bone and the Achilles tendon) for a leg injury (**Step ①b**). A pulseless arm or leg is a significant emergency that requires immediate surgical care.

- *Sensation.* This is the most useful sign. Lightly touch or squeeze the victim's toes or fingers and ask the victim what he or she feels. Loss of sensation is an early sign of nerve damage or spinal damage (**Steps ②a** and **②b**).
- *Movement.* Inability to move develops later. Check for nerve damage by asking the victim to wiggle his or her toes or fingers. If the toes or fingers are injured, do not have the victim attempt to move them (**Steps ③a** and **③b**).

5. The major blood vessels of an extremity tend to run close to the bone. Any time a bone is broken, the adjacent blood vessels are at risk of being torn by bone fragments or pinched off between the ends of the broken bone. The tissues of the arms and legs cannot survive without a continuing blood supply for more than 2 or 3 hours. In that case, seek immediate medical care.

6. Use the RICE (*rest, ice, compression, elevation*) procedures (see page 116).

7. Stabilize the injured part to prevent movement:
   - If the EMS will arrive soon, stabilize the injured part with your hands and/or against the vicitm's body until the EMS arrives.
   - If the EMS will be delayed or if you are taking the victim to medical care, use a splint to stabilize the fracture (see below).

8. Seek medical care.

▶ Splinting

Splinting an injured area helps to:
- Reduce pain
- Prevent further damage to muscle, nerves, and blood vessels
- Prevent a closed fracture from becoming an open fracture
- Reduce bleeding and swelling

Types of Splints

A <u>splint</u> is any device used to stabilize a fracture or a dislocation. Such a device can be improvised from a folded newspaper or it can be a commercial splint (eg, SAM splint). Lack of a commercial splint should never prevent you from properly stabilizing an injured extremity.

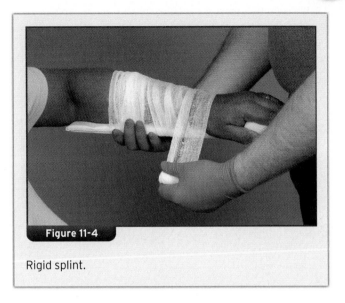

Figure 11-4

Rigid splint.

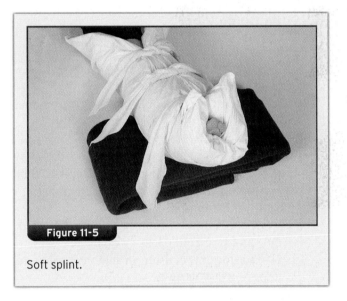

Figure 11-5

Soft splint.

A *rigid splint* is an inflexible device, such as a padded board, a piece of heavy cardboard, or a SAM splint, that is used to stabilize the extremity. It must be long enough so that it can stabilize the area above and below the fracture site **Figure 11-4**. A *soft splint*, such as a pillow or rolled blanket, is useful mainly for stabilizing fractures of the ankle **Figure 11-5**.

A *self,* or *anatomic, splint* is one in which the injured body part is tied to an uninjured part (eg, an injured finger can be tied to the adjacent finger, an injured arm to the chest, or the legs to each other) **Figure 11-6**.

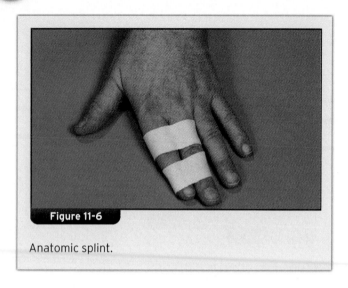

Figure 11-6

Anatomic splint.

Splinting Guidelines

The following guidelines should be used when splinting:

- Cover any open wounds with a dressing before applying a splint.
- Apply a splint only if it does not cause further pain to the victim.
- Splint the injured area in the position found.
- The splint should extend beyond the joints above and below an extremity fracture whenever possible.
- Apply splints firmly, but not so tightly that blood flow to an extremity is affected.
- Elevate the injured extremity after it is splinted.
- Apply an ice or cold pack.

To splint the lower arm using an anatomic splint, follow the steps in **Skill Drill 11-2**.

1. Use a triangular bandage to create a **sling** to support the injured arm (**Step ❶**).
2. Tie the ends of the triangular bandage and secure the sling at the elbow (**Steps ❷ₐ** and **❷ᵦ**).
3. Use a triangular bandage folded into a wide binder to secure the sling and the arm to the chest (**Step ❸**).

To apply a rigid splint to the lower arm, follow the steps in **Skill Drill 11-3**.

1. Place a splint under the injured arm in the position found. Place the hand in its normal position. A roll of gauze should be placed in the hand to maintain normal position of the hand (**Step ❶**).

2. Secure the splint with a roll of gauze or two triangular bandages folded into binders (**Step ❷**).
3. Use a triangular bandage to create a sling to support the injured arm (**Step ❸**).
4. Tie the ends of the triangular bandage and secure the sling at the elbow (**Step ❹**).
5. Use a triangular bandage folded into a wide binder to secure the sling and the splint to the chest (**Step ❺**).

To apply a soft splint to the lower arm, follow the steps in **Skill Drill 11-4**.

1. Use a rolled blanket or folded pillow to provide a splint for the injured arm in the position found (**Step ❶**).
2. Secure the splint with several triangular bandages folded into binders (**Step ❷**).
3. Use a triangular bandage to create a sling to support the injured arm (**Step ❸**).
4. Tie the ends of the triangular bandage and secure the sling at the elbow (**Steps ❹ₐ** and **❹ᵦ**).
5. Use a triangular bandage folded into a wide binder to secure the sling and the splint to the chest (**Step ❺**).

All fractures and dislocations should be stabilized before the victim is moved. When in doubt, apply a splint.

▶ Joint Injuries

A **sprain** is an injury to a joint in which the ligaments and other tissues are damaged by violent stretching or twisting. Attempts to move or use the joint increase the pain. The skin around the joint may be discolored because of bleeding from torn tissues. It often is difficult to distinguish between a severe sprain and a fracture, because their signs and symptoms are similar.

A **dislocation** occurs when a joint comes apart and stays apart with the bone ends no longer in contact. The shoulders, elbows, fingers, hips, kneecaps, and ankles are the joints most frequently affected.

Recognizing Joint Injuries

Dislocations or sprains cause signs and symptoms similar to those of a fracture:

- Deformity
- Severe pain
- Swelling
- The inability of the victim to move the injured joint

skill drill

11-2 Applying a Self (Anatomic) Splint: Lower Arm

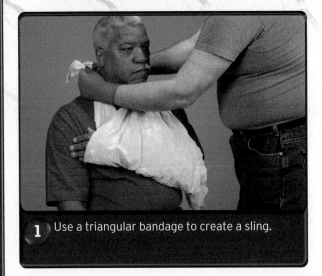

1 Use a triangular bandage to create a sling.

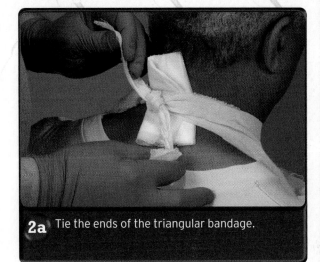

2a Tie the ends of the triangular bandage.

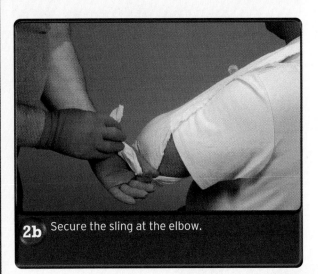

2b Secure the sling at the elbow.

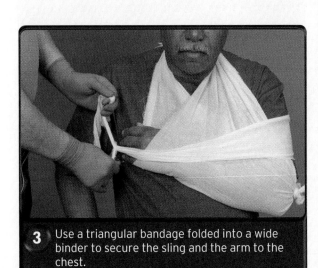

3 Use a triangular bandage folded into a wide binder to secure the sling and the arm to the chest.

skill drill

11-3   **Applying a Rigid Splint: Lower Arm**

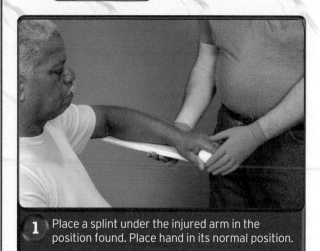

1   Place a splint under the injured arm in the position found. Place hand in its normal position.

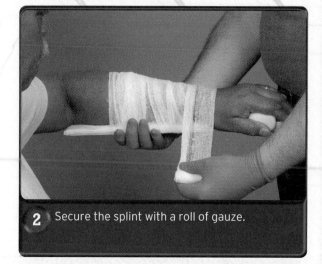

2   Secure the splint with a roll of gauze.

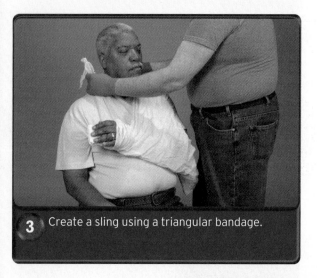

3   Create a sling using a triangular bandage.

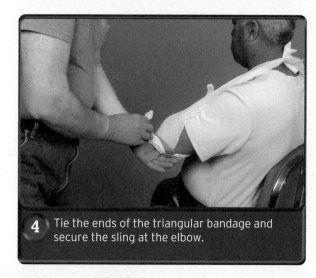

4   Tie the ends of the triangular bandage and secure the sling at the elbow.

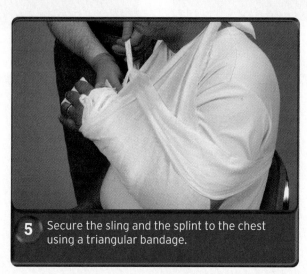

5   Secure the sling and the splint to the chest using a triangular bandage.

skill drill

11-4 | **Applying a Soft Splint: Lower Arm**

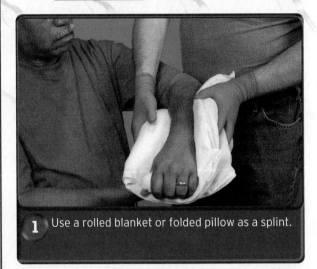

1 Use a rolled blanket or folded pillow as a splint.

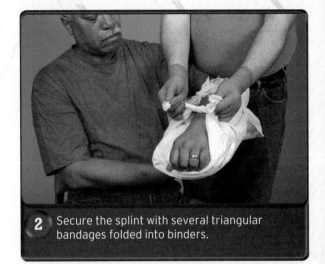

2 Secure the splint with several triangular bandages folded into binders.

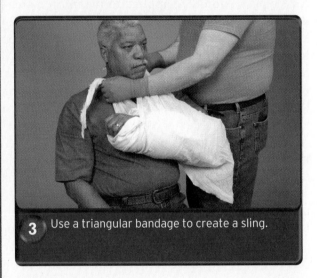

3 Use a triangular bandage to create a sling.

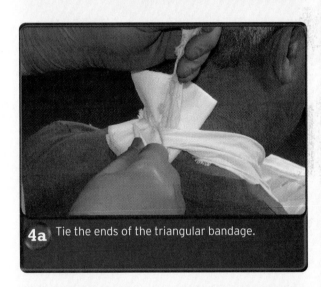

4a Tie the ends of the triangular bandage.

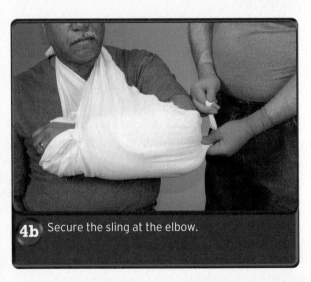

4b Secure the sling at the elbow.

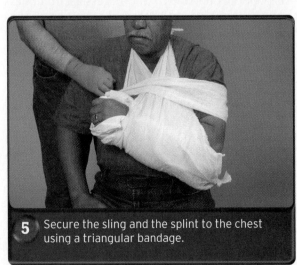

5 Secure the sling and the splint to the chest using a triangular bandage.

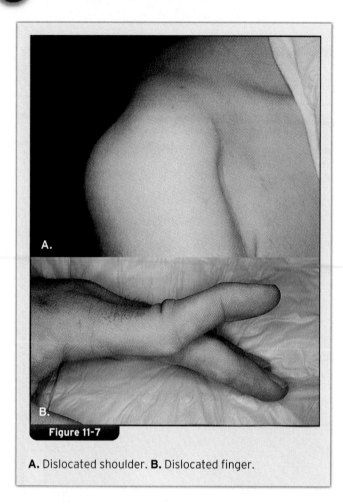

Figure 11-7

A. Dislocated shoulder. **B.** Dislocated finger.

A dislocated joint will definitely look different from an uninjured joint **Figure 11-7 A, B** .

Care for Joint Injuries

To care for a joint injury:

1. Check the CSM. If the end of the dislocated bone is pressing on nerves or blood vessels, numbness or paralysis may exist below the dislocation. Always check the pulses. If there is no pulse in the injured extremity, transport the victim to a medical care facility immediately.
2. Use the RICE procedure.
3. Use a splint to stabilize the joint in the position in which it was found.
4. Do not try to reduce the joint (put the displaced parts back into their normal positions), because damage to the nerves and blood vessels could result.
5. Seek medical care to reduce the dislocation.

▶ RICE Procedure

RICE is the acronym for the first aid procedures—*rest, ice, compression, elevation*—for bone, joint, and muscle injuries. The steps you take in the first 48 to 72 hours after such an injury can help to relieve, and even prevent, aches and pains. Treat all extremity bone, joint, and muscle injuries with the RICE procedures. In addition to RICE, fractures and dislocations should be splinted to stabilize the injured area. To perform the RICE procedure, follow the steps in **Skill Drill 11-5** .

R = Rest

Injuries heal faster if they are rested. Rest means that the victim does not use or move the injured part. Using any part of the body increases the blood circulation to that area, which can cause more swelling of an injured part. Crutches may be used to rest leg injuries.

I = Ice

An ice pack should be applied to the injured area for 20 to 30 minutes every 2 or 3 hours during the first 24 to 48 hours (**Step 1**). Skin treated with cold passes through four stages: cold, burning, aching, and numbness. When the skin becomes numb, usually in 20 to 30 minutes, remove the ice pack. After removing the ice pack, compress the injured part with an elastic bandage and keep it elevated (the "C" and "E" of RICE).

Cold constricts the blood vessels to and in the injured area, which helps to reduce the swelling and inflammation as it dulls the pain and relieves muscle spasms. Cold should be applied as soon as possible after the injury—healing time often is directly related to the amount of swelling that occurs. Heat has the opposite effect when applied to fresh injuries: it increases circulation to the area and greatly increases both the swelling and the pain.

Use either of the following methods to apply cold to an injury:

- Put crushed ice (or cubes) into a double plastic bag, hot water bottle, or wet towel. Use an elastic bandage to hold the ice pack in place. Ice bags can conform to the body's contours.
- Use a chemical cold pack, a sealed pouch that contains two chemical envelopes. Squeezing the pack mixes the chemicals, producing a chemical reaction that has a cooling effect. Although they do not cool as well as other methods, they are convenient to use when ice is not readily available. They lose

skill drill

11-5   RICE Procedure

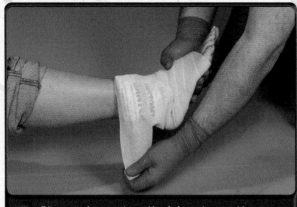

1 Place an ice pack on the injured area. Use an elastic bandage to hold the ice pack in place for 20 to 30 minutes.

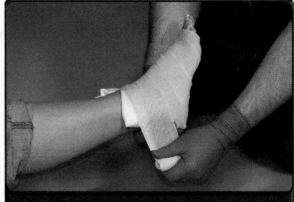

2 Remove the ice and apply a compression bandage and leave in place for 3 or 4 hours.

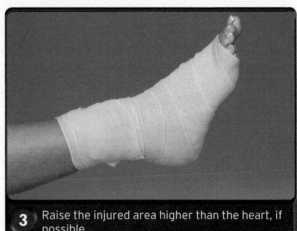

3 Raise the injured area higher than the heart, if possible.

their cooling power quickly, however, and can be used only once. Also, they may be impractical because they are expensive and can break.

> **CAUTION**
>
> DO NOT apply an ice pack for more than 20 to 30 minutes at a time. Frostbite or nerve damage can result.
>
> DO NOT apply cold if the victim has a history of circulatory disease, Raynaud's syndrome (spasms in the arteries of the extremities that reduce circulation), abnormal sensitivity to cold, or if the injured part has been frostbitten previously.
>
> DO NOT stop using an ice pack too soon. A common mistake is the early use of heat, which will result in swelling and pain. Use an ice pack three to four times a day for the first 24 hours, preferably up to 48 hours, before applying any heat. For severe injuries, using ice for up to 72 hours is recommended.

C = Compression

Compressing the injured area may squeeze some fluid and debris out of the injury site. Compression limits the ability of the skin and of other tissues to expand and reduces internal bleeding. Apply an elastic bandage to the injured area, especially the foot, ankle, knee, thigh, hand, or elbow (**Step ❷**). Fill the hollow areas such as around an ankle knob bone with padding such as a sock or washcloth before applying the elastic bandage.

Elastic bandages come in various sizes to accommodate different body areas:

- 2-inch width, used for the wrist and hand
- 3-inch width, used for the ankle, elbow, and arm
- 4- or 6-inch width, used for the ankle, knee, and leg

Start the elastic bandage several inches below the injury and wrap in an upward, overlapping (about one-half the bandage's width) spiral, starting with an even, slightly tight pressure. Gradually wrap more loosely above the injury. Stretch a new elastic bandage to about one-third its maximum length for adequate compression. Leave fingers and toes exposed so possible color change can be observed easily. Compare the toes or fingers of the injured extremity with the uninjured one. Pale skin, pain, numbness, and tingling are signs that the bandage is too tight. If any of these symptoms appear, immediately remove the elastic bandage. Leave the elastic bandage off until all the symptoms disappear, then rewrap the area, less tightly. Always wrap from below the injury and move toward the heart.

Applying compression may be the most important step in preventing swelling. The victim should wear the elastic bandage continuously for the first 18 to 24 hours (except when cold is being applied). At night, have the victim loosen, but not remove, the elastic bandage.

For an ankle injury, place a horseshoe-shaped pad around the ankle knob bone and secure with the elastic bandage. The pad will help compress the soft tissues rather than just the bones. Wrap the bandage tightest nearest the toes and loosest above the ankle. It should be tight enough to decrease swelling but not tight enough to inhibit blood flow. For a contusion or a strain, place a pad between the injury and the elastic bandage (see Muscle Injuries for more information).

E = Elevation

Gravity slows the return of blood to the heart from the lower parts of the body. Once fluids get to the hands or feet, they have nowhere else to go and those parts of the body swell. Elevating the injured area (**Step ❸**), in combination with ice and compression, limits circulation to that area, helps limit internal bleeding, and minimizes swelling.

It is simple to prop up an injured leg or arm to limit bleeding. Whenever possible, elevate the injured part above the level of the heart for the first 24 hours after an injury. If a fracture dislocation is suspected, do not elevate an extremity until it has been stabilized with a splint.

> **CAUTION**
>
> DO NOT apply an elastic bandage too tightly. If applied too tightly, elastic bandages will restrict circulation.

▶ Muscle Injuries

A muscle **strain**, or pulled muscle, occurs when a muscle is stretched beyond its normal range of motion and tears. A muscle **contusion**, or bruise, results from a blow to the muscle. A muscle contusion is an injury that causes a hemorrhage in or beneath the skin but does not break it. A **cramp** occurs when a muscle goes into an uncontrolled spasm.

Recognizing Muscle Injuries

Any of the following signs and symptoms may indicate a muscle strain:

- Sharp pain
- Extreme tenderness when the area is touched
- Cavity, indentation, or bump that can be felt or seen

- Severe weakness and loss of function of the injured part
- Stiffness and pain when the victim moves the muscle

Any of the following signs and symptoms may occur in a muscle contusion:

- Swelling
- Pain and tenderness
- Black-and-blue mark appearing hours later

The signs of a muscle cramp include the following:

- Uncontrolled spasm
- Pain
- Restriction or loss of movement
- Muscle is usually hard to touch

Care for Muscle Injuries

To care for muscle strains and contusions:

1. Rest the affected muscle(s).
2. Apply an ice or cold pack to the affected area.

A number of treatments for cramps are available. Try one or more of the following:

1. Have the victim gently stretch the affected muscle. Because a muscle cramp is an uncontrolled muscle contraction or spasm, a gradual lengthening of the muscle may help lengthen the muscle fibers and relieve the cramp.
2. Relax the muscle by applying pressure to it.
3. Apply ice to the cramped muscle to make it relax, unless you are in a cold environment.
4. Pinch the upper lip hard (an acupressure technique) to reduce calf-muscle cramping.

> **CAUTION**
>
> DO NOT give salt tablets to a person with muscle cramps. They can cause stomach irritation, nausea, and vomiting.
>
> DO NOT massage or rub the affected muscle. This only causes more pain and does not relieve the cramping.

▶ Other Injuries

Blood Under a Nail

When a fingernail has been crushed, blood collects under the nail. This condition usually is very painful because of the pressure of the blood pressing against the nail **Figure 11-8** .

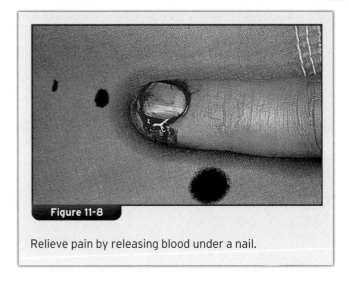

Figure 11-8

Relieve pain by releasing blood under a nail.

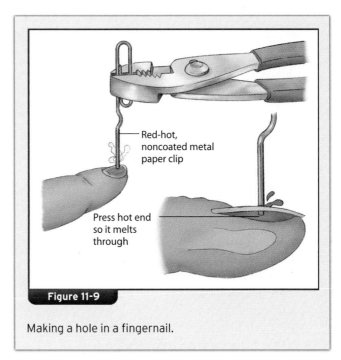

Red-hot, noncoated metal paper clip

Press hot end so it melts through

Figure 11-9

Making a hole in a fingernail.

Care for Blood Under a Nail

1. Immerse the finger in ice water or apply an ice pack with the hand elevated.
2. By using one of the following methods, relieve the pressure under the injured nail:
   - Straighten the end of a metal (noncoated) paper clip or use the blunt (eye) end of a sewing needle. Hold the paper clip or needle with pliers and use a match or cigarette lighter to heat it until the metal is red hot. Press the glowing end of the paper clip or needle against the nail until it melts through. Little pressure is needed. The nail has no nerves, so this can be a painless procedure. The nailbed below the nail does contain nerves. **Figure 11-9** .

- Using a rotary action, drill through the nail with the sharp point of a knife.

3. Apply a dressing to absorb the draining blood and to protect the injured nail.

Ring Strangulation

Sometimes a finger is so swollen that a ring cannot be removed. Ring strangulation can be a serious problem if it cuts off circulation long enough. Try one or more of the following methods to remove a ring:

- Lubricate the finger with grease, oil, butter, petroleum jelly, or some other slippery substance, and then try to remove the ring.
- Immerse the finger in cold water or apply an ice pack for several minutes to reduce the swelling.
- Massage the finger from the tip to the hand to move the swelling; lubricate the finger again and try removing the ring.
- If the ring cannot be removed, immediately transport the victim to the emergency room. If prompt transportation is not available, call 9-1-1. They can use a ring-cutter to remove the ring when all else fails.

▶ Bone Injuries

What to Look For

Fractures (broken bones)
- DOTS (deformity, open wound, tenderness, swelling)
- Inability to use injured part normally
- Grating or grinding sensation felt or heard
- Victim heard or felt bone snap

What to Do

1. Expose and examine the injury site.
2. Bandage any open wound.
3. Splint the injured area.
4. Apply ice or cold pack.
5. Seek medical care: Depending on the severity, call 9-1-1 or transport to medical care.

▶ Joint Injuries

What to Look For

Dislocation or sprain
- Deformity
- Pain
- Swelling
- Inability to use injured part normally

What to Do

Dislocation
1. Expose and examine the injury site.
2. Splint the injured area.
3. Apply ice or cold pack.
4. Seek medical care.
Sprain
1. Use RICE procedures.

▶ Muscle Injuries

What to Look For

Strain
- Sharp pain
- Extreme tenderness when area is touched
- Indentation or bump
- Weakness and loss of function of injured area
- Stiffness and pain when victim moves the muscle

Contusion
- Pain and tenderness
- Swelling
- Bruise on injured area

Cramp
- Uncontrolled spasm
- Pain
- Restriction or loss of movement

What to Do

1. Use RICE procedures.

1. Use RICE procedures.

1. Stretch and/or apply direct pressure to the affected muscle.

prep kit

▶ Ready for Review

- Fractures are open or closed. Open fractures have a wound resulting from a bone protruding through the skin or an external object broke the skin while breaking the underlying bone.
- A splint is a device used to stabilize a fracture or dislocation.
- Splints can be improvised (eg, folded newspaper) or commercial (eg, SAM splint). They may also be rigid (eg, SAM splint) or soft (eg, pillow).
- A self splint is one in which the injured part is tied to an uninjured body part (eg, taping two fingers together).
- When in doubt, apply a splint.
- The injured part should, in most cases, be splinted in the position found.
- The acronym DOTS is helpful in remembering what to look and feel for during a physical exam.
- An injured extremity with a suspected fracture or dislocation should be examined for circulation, sensation, and movement.
- RICE is the acronym for *rest, ice, compression,* and *elevation,* which should be used for most fractures, dislocations, sprains, and strains.
- Sprains and dislocations are both joint injuries. A fracture is a break in a bone. Muscle injuries include: strain, contusion or bruise, and a cramp.

▶ Vital Vocabulary

<u>closed fracture</u> A fracture in which there is no wound in the overlaying skin.

<u>contusion</u> A bruise; results from a blow to the muscle.

<u>cramp</u> A painful spasm, usually of the muscle.

<u>dislocation</u> Occurs when a joint comes apart and stays apart with the bone ends no longer in contact.

<u>fracture</u> A break or a crack in a bone.

<u>open fracture</u> A fracture exposed to the exterior; an open wound lies over the fracture.

<u>sling</u> Any bandage or material that helps support the weight of an injured upper extremity.

<u>splint</u> Any support used to immobilize a fracture or restrict movement of a part.

<u>sprain</u> A trauma to a joint that injures the ligaments.

<u>strain</u> Known as a pulled muscle; occurs when a muscle is stretched beyond its normal range of motion and tears.

▶ Assessment in Action

You and several friends are playing a friendly game of basketball on a warm summer day in the driveway. One of your teammates after going up for a shot comes down and twists his ankle. He is sitting on the concrete driveway holding his ankle and complaining about the pain. *Directions:* Circle *Yes* if you agree with the statement and *No* if you disagree.

Yes No **1.** The ankle could be either sprained or fractured.

Yes No **2.** An ankle injury will benefit from a RICE treatment.

Yes No **3.** Shortly after the injury apply heat to increase blood circulation to the injured area.

Yes No **4.** When using an ice pack, do not leave it on the injured area for longer than 20 to 30 minutes.

Answers: **1.** Yes; **2.** Yes; **3.** No; **4.** Yes

▶ Check Your Knowledge

Directions: Circle *Yes* if you agree with the statement and *No* if you disagree.

Yes No **1.** For a suspected arm or leg fracture, check for blood flow and nerve responses.

Yes No **2.** Apply cold on a suspected fracture.

Yes No **3.** A splint can help stabilize (keep in place) a fracture.

Yes No **4.** The letters RICE represent the treatment that can be used for musculoskeletal injuries.

Yes No **5.** When using an ice pack, place it over the injury and hold it in place with an elastic bandage.

Yes No **6.** Applying heat too soon to the injury is a common mistake.

Yes No **7.** An elastic bandage, if used correctly, can help control swelling in a joint.

Yes No **8.** Give salt tablets to a person suffering muscle cramps.

Yes No **9.** Apply heat initially to a muscle injury.

Yes No **10.** A pillow can serve as a splint.

Answers: **1.** Yes; **2.** Yes; **3.** Yes; **4.** Yes; **5.** Yes; **6.** Yes; **7.** Yes; **8.** No; **9.** No; **10.** Yes

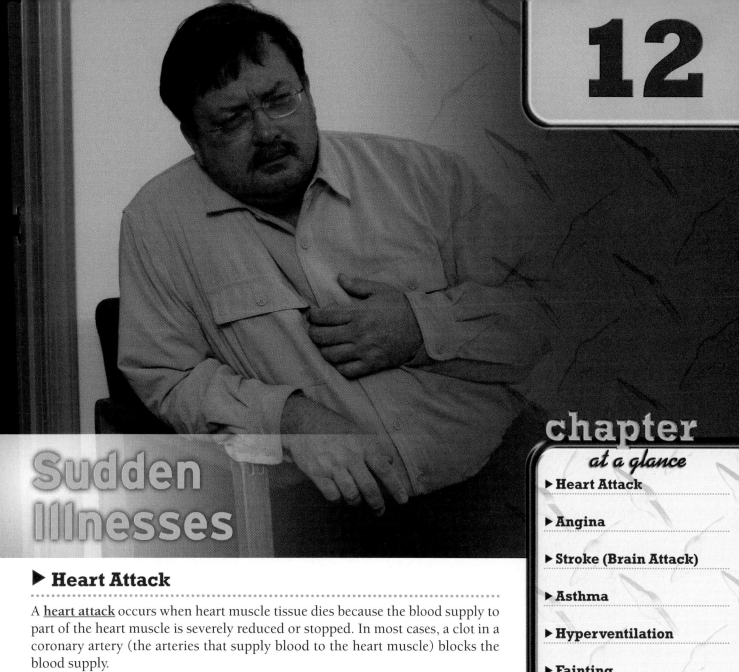

Sudden Illnesses

▶ Heart Attack

A <u>heart attack</u> occurs when heart muscle tissue dies because the blood supply to part of the heart muscle is severely reduced or stopped. In most cases, a clot in a coronary artery (the arteries that supply blood to the heart muscle) blocks the blood supply.

Recognizing a Heart Attack

It is difficult to determine if a victim is having a heart attack. Because medical care at the onset of a heart attack is vital to the victim's survival and the quality of recovery, if you suspect a heart attack for any reason, seek medical care at once.

Possible signs and symptoms of a heart attack include:

- Uncomfortable pressure, fullness, squeezing, or pain in the center of the chest that lasts more than a few minutes or that goes away and comes back
- Pain spreading to the shoulders, neck, or arms
- Dizziness, fainting, sweating, nausea
- Shortness of breath

Not all these warning signs occur in every heart attack. Many victims will deny that they are experiencing something as serious as a heart attack. Delay can seriously increase the risk of major damage. Insist on taking prompt action.

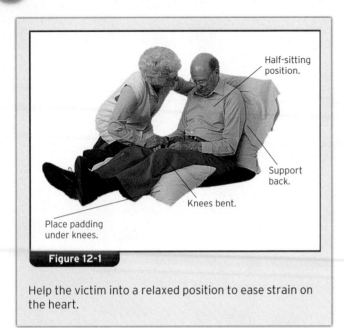

Figure 12-1

Help the victim into a relaxed position to ease strain on the heart.

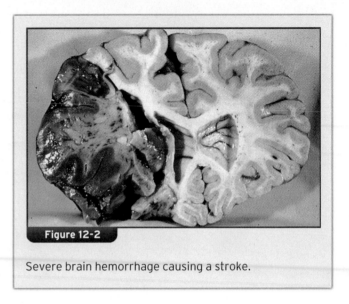

Figure 12-2

Severe brain hemorrhage causing a stroke.

Care for a Heart Attack

To care for a heart attack:

1. Call 9-1-1 or get to the nearest hospital emergency department with 24-hour emergency cardiac care.
2. Monitor breathing.
3. Help the victim to the most comfortable position, usually sitting with legs up and bent at the knees **Figure 12-1** . Loosen clothing around the neck and midriff. Be calm and reassuring.
4. If the victim is alert, able to swallow, and not allergic to aspirin, give one adult aspirin or two to four chewable children's aspirin.
5. Determine if the victim is using nitroglycerin. Nitroglycerin tablets or spray under the tongue or nitroglycerin ointment on the skin may relieve chest pain. Nitroglycerin dilates the coronary arteries, which increases blood flow to the heart muscle, and lowers blood pressure and dilates the veins, which decreases the work of the heart and the heart muscle's need for oxygen. *Caution:* Because nitroglycerin lowers blood pressure, the victim should sit or lie down once it is taken.
6. If the victim is unresponsive, check breathing and start CPR, if needed.

▶ Angina

Chest pain called *angina pectoris* can result from coronary heart disease just as a heart attack does. **Angina** happens when the heart muscle does not get as much blood as it needs (which means a lack of oxygen). Angina is brought on by physical exertion, exposure to cold, emotional stress, or the ingestion of food.

Recognizing Angina

It can be difficult to differentiate a heart attack from angina, even for physicians. The signs are similar to those of a heart attack, but seldom last longer than 10 minutes and almost always are relieved by nitroglycerin. In contrast, chest pain from a heart attack is as likely to happen at rest as during activity; the pain lasts longer than 10 minutes and is not relieved by nitroglycerin.

Care for Angina

To care for angina:

1. Have the victim rest.
2. If the victim has nitroglycerin, help him or her use it.
3. If the pain continues beyond 10 minutes, suspect a heart attack and call 9-1-1.

▶ Stroke (Brain Attack)

A **stroke**, also referred to as a *brain attack* or *cerebrovascular accident (CVA)*, occurs when blood vessels that deliver oxygen-rich blood to the brain rupture or become plugged, so part of the brain does not get the blood flow it needs **Figure 12-2** and **Figure 12-3** . Deprived of oxygen-rich blood, nerve cells in the affected area of the brain cannot function and die within minutes. Because dead brain cells are not replaced, the devastating effects of a stroke often are permanent.

Transient ischemic attacks (TIAs) are closely associated with strokes. Because TIAs have many of the same signs and symptoms, they often are confused with strokes.

Heart Attack

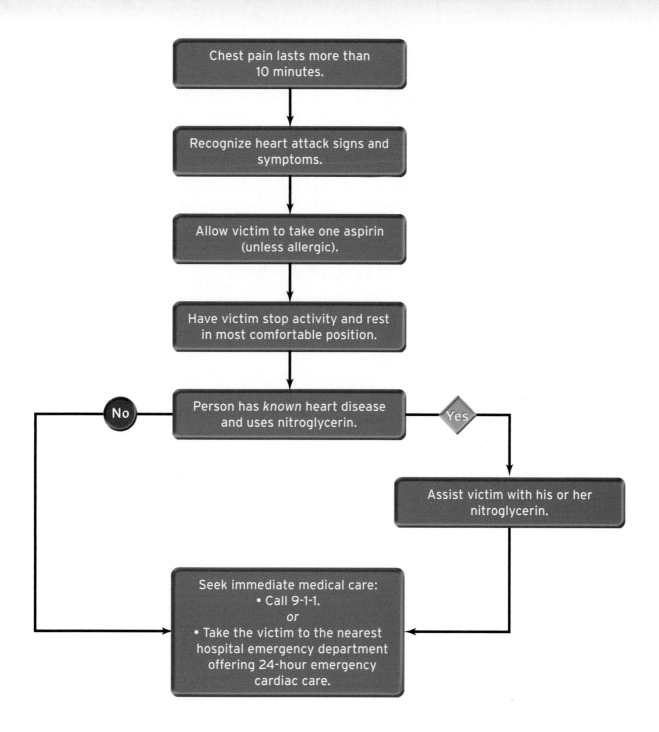

Chest pain lasts more than 10 minutes.

Recognize heart attack signs and symptoms.

Allow victim to take one aspirin (unless allergic).

Have victim stop activity and rest in most comfortable position.

Person has *known* heart disease and uses nitroglycerin.

No

Yes

Assist victim with his or her nitroglycerin.

Seek immediate medical care:
• Call 9-1-1.
or
• Take the victim to the nearest hospital emergency department offering 24-hour emergency cardiac care.

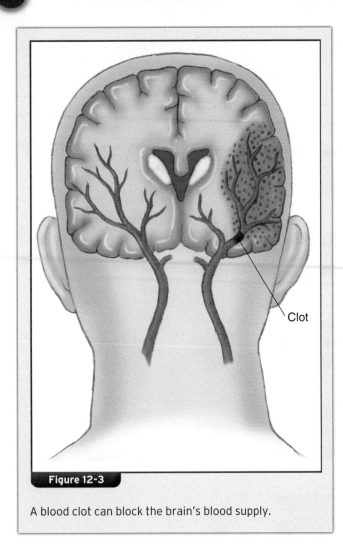

Figure 12-3

A blood clot can block the brain's blood supply.

The main difference between a TIA and a stroke is that the symptoms of TIA are transient, lasting from several minutes (75% last less than 5 minutes) to several hours, with a return to normal neurologic function. TIAs are "mini-strokes." A TIA should be considered a serious warning sign of a potential stroke—about one-third of all TIA cases will suffer a stroke within 2 to 5 years after their first TIA. Any signs and symptoms of a TIA should be reported to a physician.

Recognizing Stroke

The signs of stroke include the following:
- Weakness, numbness, or paralysis of the face, an arm, or a leg on one side of the body **Figure 12-4 A, B**.
- Blurred or decreased vision, especially in one eye
- Problems speaking or understanding
- Dizziness or loss of balance
- Sudden, severe, and unexplained headache
- Deviation of the pupils of the eyes from PEARL (Pupils Equal And Reactive to Light), which may mean the brain is being affected by lack of oxygen

Care for Stroke

First aid for a stroke victim is limited to supportive care:
1. If victim is unresponsive, check for breathing.
2. Call 9-1-1.
3. If the victim is responsive, lay the victim down with the head and shoulders slightly elevated to reduce blood pressure on the brain.
4. Place an unresponsive breathing victim in the recovery position, which is on the side (to keep the airway open and to permit secretions and vomit to drain from the mouth).

CAUTION

DO NOT give a stroke victim anything to drink or eat. The throat may be paralyzed, which restricts swallowing.

▶ Asthma

Asthma is a condition in which air passages narrow and mucus builds up, resulting in poor oxygen exchange. It can be triggered by such things as an allergy, cold exposure, smoke, strong odors, exercise, and air pollution, among other triggers.

Recognizing Asthma

The signs of asthma include the following:
- Coughing
- Cyanosis (bluish skin color)
- Inability to speak in complete sentences without pausing for breath
- Nostrils flaring with each breath
- Difficulty breathing including wheezing (high-pitched whistling sound during breathing)

Care for Asthma

To care for a victim with asthma:
1. Keep the victim in a comfortable upright position that makes it easier to breathe.
2. Monitor breathing.
3. Ask the victim about any asthma medication he or she may be using **Figure 12-5**. Most asthma sufferers will have some form of asthma medication, usually administered through physician-prescribed, handheld inhalers.
4. If the victim does not respond well to the inhaled medication or is having an extreme asthma attack (known as *status asthmaticus*), call 9-1-1 immediately.

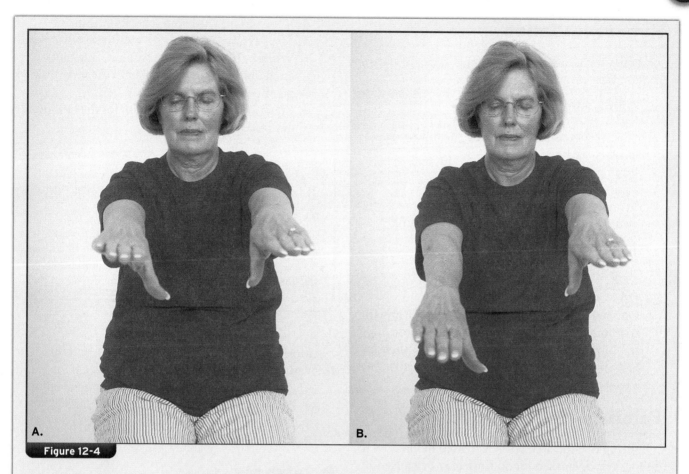

Figure 12-4

One-sided weakness (stroke test). **A.** Arms straight out. **B.** One arm dropped (see FYI box on this page, for details).

FYI

Los Angeles Stroke Screen

Los Angeles paramedics use a proven method for quickly identifying stroke victims, and so can first aiders. When you suspect a stroke, apply these three simple tests for one-side paralysis:

1. *Arm strength (both arms):* person closes eyes and holds both arms out with palms down. Slowly count to five. If one arm does not move and the other drifts down, suspect a stroke.

2. *Facial smile:* person smiles or shows teeth. If one side of face does not move as well as the other side, suspect a stroke.

3. *Hand grip (both hands):* person grips two of your fingers at the same time. If grip strength is not equal, suspect a stroke.

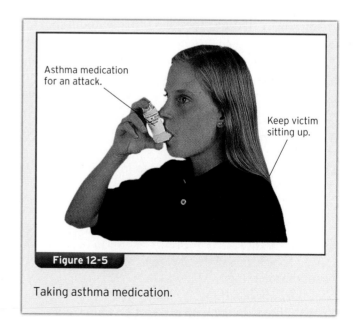

Asthma medication for an attack.

Keep victim sitting up.

Figure 12-5

Taking asthma medication.

▶ Hyperventilation

<u>Hyperventilation</u> is fast, deep breathing that can be caused by emotional stress, anxiety, and medical conditions.

Recognizing Hyperventilation

The signs of hyperventilation include the following:
- Dizziness or lightheadedness
- Numbness
- Tingling of the hands and feet
- Shortness of breath
- Breathing rates faster than 40 times per minute

Care for Hyperventilation

To care for hyperventilation:
1. Calm and reassure the victim.
2. Encourage the victim to breathe slowly, using the abdominal muscles. Inhale through the nose, hold the full inhalation for several seconds, then exhale slowly. Do NOT have the victim breathe into a paper bag.

▶ Fainting

Most <u>fainting</u> is associated with decreased blood flow to the brain. The decreased blood flow may be caused by low blood sugar (hypoglycemia), slow heart rate (vagal reaction, in which the vagus nerve, which slows the heart rate, is overstimulated by fright, anxiety, drugs, or fatigue), heart-rhythm disturbances, dehydration, heat exhaustion, anemia, or bleeding.

Sitting or standing for a long time without moving, especially in a hot environment, can cause blood to pool in dilated vessels. This results in a loss of effective circulating blood volume, and blood pressure drops. As the blood flow to the brain decreases, the person loses consciousness and collapses.

Recognizing Fainting

The signs of fainting include the following:
- Sudden, brief unresponsiveness
- Pale skin
- Sweating

Care for Fainting

To care for fainting:
1. Check breathing.
2. Raise the victim's legs 6 to 12 inches
3. Loosen tight clothing and belts.

4. If the victim has fallen, check for injuries.
5. After recovery, have the victim sit for a while. When he or she is able to swallow, give cool, sweetened liquids to drink, and help the victim slowly regain an upright posture.
6. Fresh air and a cold, wet cloth for the face usually aid recovery.

CAUTION

DO NOT splash or pour water on the victim's face.

DO NOT use smelling salts or ammonia inhalants.

DO NOT slap the victim's face in an attempt to revive him or her.

DO NOT give the victim anything to drink until he or she has fully recovered and can swallow.

Most fainting episodes are not serious, and the victim recovers quickly. Seek medical care, however, if the victim:
- Has had repeated attacks of unresponsiveness
- Does not quickly regain responsiveness
- Loses responsiveness while sitting or lying down
- Faints for no apparent reason

▶ Seizures

A <u>seizure</u> results from an abnormal stimulation of the brain's cells. A variety of medical conditions can lead to seizures, including the following:
- Epilepsy
- Heatstroke
- Poisoning
- Electric shock
- Hypoglycemia
- High fever in children
- Brain injury, tumor, or stroke
- Alcohol withdrawal, drug abuse/overdose

Epilepsy is not a mental illness, and it is not a sign of low intelligence. It also is not contagious. Between seizures, a person with epilepsy functions normally.

Recognizing Seizure

The signs of a seizure will vary depending on the type of seizure and can include the following:
- Sudden falling
- Unresponsiveness
- Rigid body and arching of the back
- Jerky muscle movement

Fainting

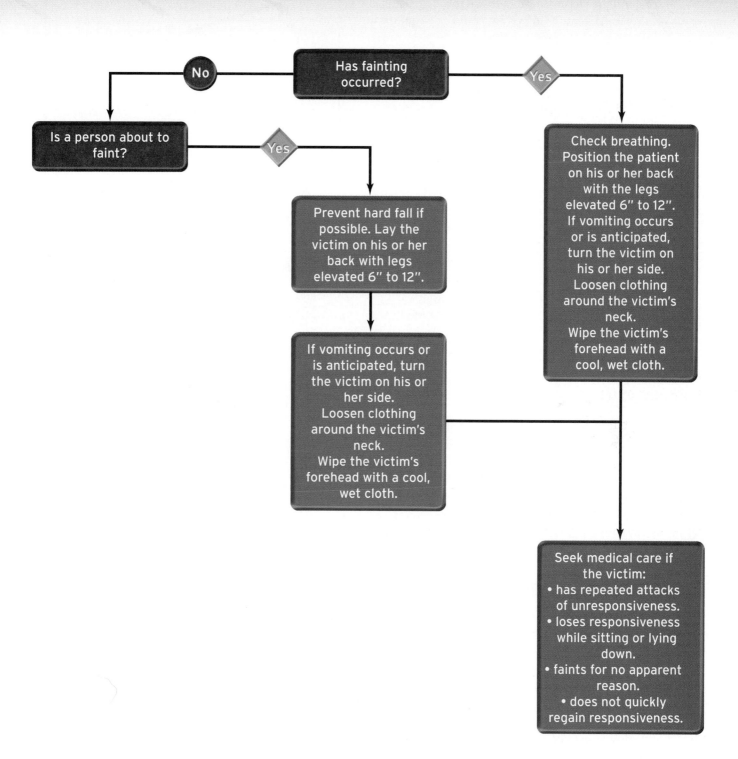

Has fainting occurred?

No

Yes

Is a person about to faint?

Yes

Prevent hard fall if possible. Lay the victim on his or her back with legs elevated 6" to 12".

If vomiting occurs or is anticipated, turn the victim on his or her side.
Loosen clothing around the victim's neck.
Wipe the victim's forehead with a cool, wet cloth.

Check breathing.
Position the patient on his or her back with the legs elevated 6" to 12".
If vomiting occurs or is anticipated, turn the victim on his or her side.
Loosen clothing around the victim's neck.
Wipe the victim's forehead with a cool, wet cloth.

Seek medical care if the victim:
• has repeated attacks of unresponsiveness.
• loses responsiveness while sitting or lying down.
• faints for no apparent reason.
• does not quickly regain responsiveness.

Care for a Seizure

The Epilepsy Foundation lists the following first aid procedures for seizures:

1. Cushion the victim's head (a rolled towel or jacket works well); remove items that could cause injury if the person bumped into them.
2. Loosen any tight clothing, especially around the neck.
3. Roll the victim onto his or her side.
4. As the seizure ends, offer your help. Most seizures in people with epilepsy are not medical emergencies. They end after a minute or two without harm and usually do not require medical care.
5. Call 9-1-1 if any of the following exists:
   - A seizure occurs in someone who is not known to have epilepsy (eg, there is no "epilepsy" or "seizure disorder" identification). It could be a sign of serious illness.
   - A seizure lasts longer than 5 minutes.
   - The victim is slow to recover, has a second seizure, or has difficulty breathing afterward.
   - The victim is pregnant or has another medical condition.
   - There are any signs of injury or illnesses.

CAUTION

DO NOT give the victim anything to eat or drink.

DO NOT put anything between the victim's teeth.

DO NOT restrain the victim.

DO NOT splash or pour water on the victim's face.

DO NOT move the victim to another place (unless it is the only way to protect the victim from injury).

▶ Diabetic Emergencies

<u>Diabetes</u> is a condition in which insulin, a hormone produced by the pancreas that helps the body use the energy in food, is either lacking or ineffective. Insulin is needed to take sugar from the blood and carry it into the cells to be used. When sugar remains in the blood, the body cells must rely on fat as fuel. Blood sugar (glucose) is a major body fuel, and when it cannot be used, it builds up in the blood, overflows into the urine, and passes out of the body unused, so the body loses an important source of fuel. Diabetes then develops. Diabetes is not contagious.

There are two types of diabetes:
- *Type I* (formerly called *juvenile-onset* or *insulin-dependent diabetes*): Type I diabetics require exter-

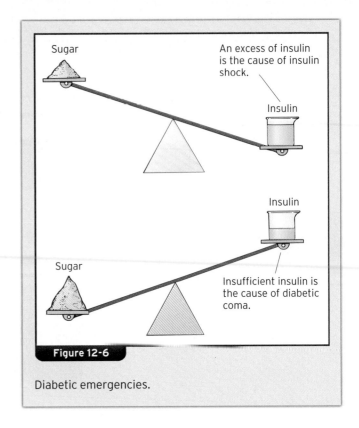

Figure 12-6

Diabetic emergencies.

nal (not made by the body) insulin to allow sugar to pass from the blood into cells. When deprived of external insulin, the diabetic becomes quite ill.
- *Type II* (formerly called *adult-onset* or *non-insulin-dependent diabetes*): Type II diabetics tend to be overweight. They are not dependent on external insulin to allow sugar into cells. However, if their insulin level is low, the lack of sugar in the cells increases sugar production and sugar in the blood to very high levels. That causes glucose to spill into the urine, drawing fluid with it, resulting in dehydration.

The body is continuously balancing sugar and insulin. Too much insulin and not enough sugar leads to low blood sugar, and possibly insulin shock. Too much sugar and not enough insulin leads to high blood sugar, and possibly diabetic coma **Figure 12-6**.

Recognizing Low Blood Sugar

Very low blood sugar, called <u>hypoglycemia</u>, is sometimes referred to as an *insulin reaction*. This condition can be caused by too much insulin, too little or delayed food, exercise, alcohol, or any combination of these factors.

The American Diabetes Association lists the following signs and symptoms of insulin reaction and hypoglycemia as diabetic emergencies requiring first aid:
- Sudden onset
- Staggering, poor coordination

Seizures

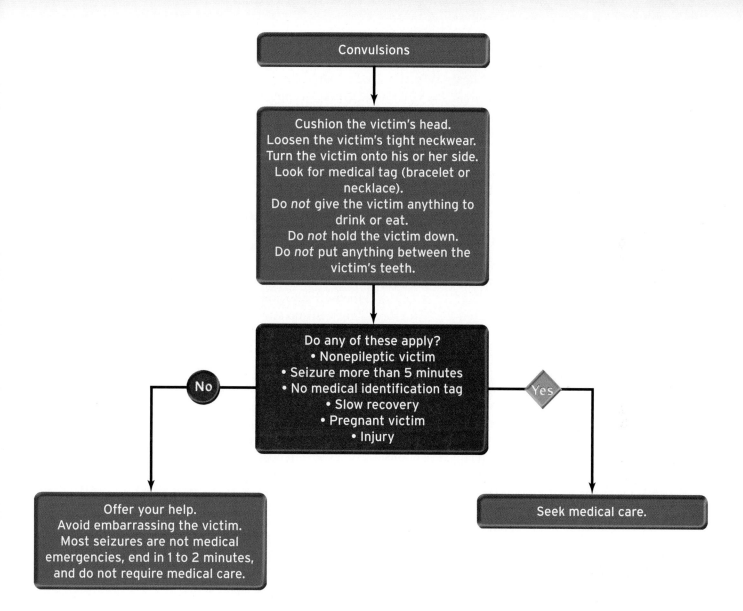

Convulsions

Cushion the victim's head.
Loosen the victim's tight neckwear.
Turn the victim onto his or her side.
Look for medical tag (bracelet or necklace).
Do *not* give the victim anything to drink or eat.
Do *not* hold the victim down.
Do *not* put anything between the victim's teeth.

Do any of these apply?
- Nonepileptic victim
- Seizure more than 5 minutes
- No medical identification tag
- Slow recovery
- Pregnant victim
- Injury

No

Yes

Offer your help.
Avoid embarrassing the victim.
Most seizures are not medical emergencies, end in 1 to 2 minutes, and do not require medical care.

Seek medical care.

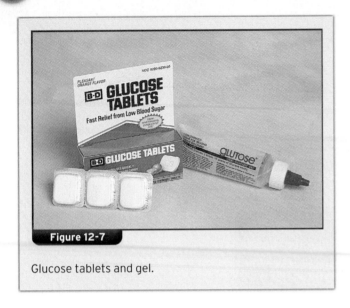

Figure 12-7

Glucose tablets and gel.

- Anger, bad temper
- Pale color
- Confusion, disorientation
- Sudden hunger
- Excessive sweating
- Trembling
- Eventual unresponsiveness

Care for Low Blood Sugar

Use the "Rule of 15s" for giving sugar if the victim is a known diabetic, mental status is changed, and is awake to swallow:

1. Give 15 grams of sugar (eg, two large teaspoons or lumps of sugar, or one-half can of regular soda, 4 oz. of orange juice, two to five glucose tablets, or one tube of glucose gel) **Figure 12-7** .
2. Wait 15 minutes.
3. If no improvement, give 15 more grams of sugar (carbohydrate).
4. If no improvement, seek immediate medical care.

Recognizing High Blood Sugar

<u>Hyperglycemia</u> is the opposite of hypoglycemia. Hyperglycemia occurs when the body has too much sugar in the blood. This condition may be caused by insufficient insulin, overeating, inactivity, illness, stress, or a combination of these factors. If severe hyperglycemia persists, it can lead to diabetic coma.

The American Diabetes Association lists the following signs and symptoms of diabetic coma and hyperglycemia as diabetic emergencies requiring first aid:

- Gradual onset
- Drowsiness

- Extreme thirst
- Very frequent urination
- Flushed skin
- Vomiting
- Fruity breath odor
- Heavy breathing
- Eventual unresponsiveness

Care for High Blood Sugar

To care for a diabetic with high blood sugar (hyperglycemia):

1. If you are uncertain whether the victim has high or low blood-sugar level, give the person food or drink containing sugar.
2. If you do not see improvement in 15 minutes, seek medical care.

▶ Emergencies During Pregnancy

Most pregnancies are normal and occur without complications. However, sometimes problems do arise and medical care is required. It is essential that you remain calm, focused, and considerate of the mother during this unforeseen and stressful situation.

Recognizing Emergencies During Pregnancy

Immediately notify a doctor to report the following signs and symptoms in a pregnant woman:

- Vaginal bleeding
- Cramps in lower abdomen
- Swelling of the face or fingers
- Severe continuous headache
- Dizziness or fainting
- Blurring of vision or seeing spots
- Uncontrollable vomiting

Care for Pregnancy Emergencies

If the victim is experiencing vaginal bleeding or abdominal pain:

1. Keep the woman quiet, warm, and on her left side.
2. Have victim or another woman place a sanitary napkin or any sterile or clean pad over the opening of the vagina.
3. Have victim or another woman replace, but save, any blood-soaked pads and all tissues that are passed. Send this with the woman to medical help for examination by the physician.
4. Seek medical care immediately.

If the victim has injuries to her lower abdomen:

1. Keep the woman quiet, warm, and on her left side.
2. Monitor breathing.
3. Seek medical care.

Diabetic Emergencies

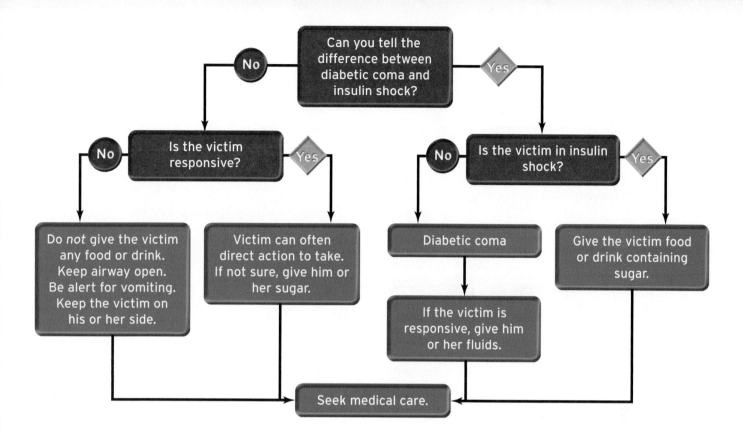

Can you tell the difference between diabetic coma and insulin shock?

No — Is the victim responsive?
- No: Do *not* give the victim any food or drink. Keep airway open. Be alert for vomiting. Keep the victim on his or her side.
- Yes: Victim can often direct action to take. If not sure, give him or her sugar.

Yes — Is the victim in insulin shock?
- No: Diabetic coma → If the victim is responsive, give him or her fluids.
- Yes: Give the victim food or drink containing sugar.

Seek medical care.

▶ Heart Attack

What to Look For

- Chest pressure, squeezing, or pain
- Pain spreading to shoulders, neck, jaw, or arms
- Dizziness, sweating, nausea
- Shortness of breath

What to Do

1. Help victim take his or her prescribed medication.
2. Call 9-1-1.
3. Help victim into a comfortable position.
4. Give one adult or two to four children's aspirin.
5. Monitor breathing.

▶ Angina

What to Look For

- Chest pain similar to a heart attack
- Pain seldom lasts longer than 10 minutes

What to Do

1. Have victim rest.
2. If victim has his or her own nitroglycerin, help the victim use it.
3. If pain continues beyond 10 minutes, suspect a heart attack and call 9-1-1.

▶ Stroke

What to Look For

- Sudden weakness or numbness of the face, an arm, or a leg on one side of the body
- Blurred or decreased vision
- Problems speaking
- Dizziness or loss of balance
- Sudden, severe headache

What to Do

1. Call 9-1-1.
2. If responsive, help victim into a comfortable position with head and shoulders slightly raised.
3. If unresponsive, move onto his or her side.

▶ Breathing Difficulty

What to Look For

- Abnormally fast or slow breathing
- Abnormally deep or shallow breathing
- Noisy breathing
- Bluish lips
- Need to pause while speaking to catch breath

What to Do

Unknown reason
1. Help victim into a comfortable position.
2. Call 9-1-1.

Asthma attack
1. Help victim into a comfortable position.
2. Help victim use inhaler.
3. Call 9-1-1 if victim does not improve.

Hyperventilating
1. Encourage victim to inhale, hold breath a few seconds, then exhale.
2. Call 9-1-1 if condition does not improve.

▶ Fainting

What to Look For

- Sudden, brief unresponsiveness
- Pale skin
- Sweating

What to Do

1. Check breathing.
2. Check for injuries if victim fell.
3. Raise feet 6 to 12 inches.
4. Call 9-1-1 if needed.

▶ Seizures

What to Look For

- Sudden falling
- Unresponsiveness
- Rigid body and arching of back
- Jerky muscle movement

What to Do

1. Prevent injury.
2. Loosen any tight clothing.
3. Roll victim onto his or her side.
4. Call 9-1-1 if needed.

▶ Diabetic Emergencies

What to Look For

Low blood sugar
- Develops very quickly
- Anger, bad temper
- Hunger
- Pale, sweaty skin

High blood sugar
- Develops gradually
- Thirst
- Frequent urination
- Fruity, sweet breath odor
- Warm and dry skin

What to Do

1. If uncertain about high or low sugar level, give sugar.
2. Repeat in 15 minutes if no improvement.
3. Call 9-1-1 if conditions do not improve.

▶ Pregnancy Emergencies

What to Look For

- Vaginal bleeding
- Cramps in lower abdomen
- Swelling of face or fingers
- Severe continuous headache
- Dizziness or fainting
- Blurring of vision or seeing spots
- Uncontrollable vomiting

What to Do

Vaginal bleeding or abdominal pain or injury

1. Keep victim warm.
2. For vaginal bleeding, place sanitary napkin or sterile or clean pad over opening of vagina.
3. Send blood-soaked pad and tissues with victim to medical care.
4. Seek medical care.

prep kit

▶ Ready for Review

- A heart attack occurs when the heart muscle tissue dies because its blood supply is reduced or stopped.
- Angina can result from coronary heart disease just as a heart attack does.
- A stroke occurs when part of the blood flow to the brain is suddenly cut off.
- Asthma is a chronic, inflammatory lung disease characterized by repeated breathing problems.
- Fainting is a sudden brief loss of responsiveness not associated with a head injury.
- A seizure results from an abnormal stimulation of the brain's cells causing uncontrollable muscle movements.
- Diabetes is a condition in which insulin is lacking or ineffective.
- If a woman experiences vaginal bleeding late in her pregnancy, it usually constitutes an emergency.

▶ Vital Vocabulary

angina When the heart muscle does not get as much blood as it needs (which means a lack of oxygen).

asthma A condition marked by recurrent attacks of breathing difficulty, often with wheezing, due to spasmodic constriction of air passages, often as a response to allergens or to mucous plugs in the bronchioles.

diabetes A general term referring to disorders characterized by excessive urine excretion, excessive thirst, and excessive hunger.

fainting Associated with decreased blood flow to the brain.

heart attack Lay term for a condition resulting from blockage of a coronary artery and subsequent death of part of the heart muscle; an acute myocardial infarction; sometimes called a *coronary*.

hyperglycemia An abnormally increased concentration of sugar in the blood.

hyperventilation Fast, deep breathing that can be caused by emotional stress, anxiety, and medical conditions.

hypoglycemia An abnormally diminished concentration of sugar in the blood.

seizure A sudden attack or recurrence of a disease; a convulsion; an attack of epilepsy.

stroke A brain injury due to blockage of blood flow causing permanent damage.

▶ Assessment in Action

Your 60-year-old father complains about chest pain. He says that it started about an hour ago and has not let up. He is sure that it is just a little indigestion and feels silly about talking about it. He says the pain feels like "something pressing on my chest," and he feels nauseous.

Directions: Circle *Yes* if you agree with the statement and *No* if you disagree.

Yes   No   1. Have him lie down for 30 minutes to see if the pain stops.

Yes   No   2. You suspect a heart attack.

Yes   No   3. Help him take an aspirin, and call 9-1-1.

Yes   No   4. Heart attack victims often resist the idea that they need medical care.

Answers: 1. No; 2. Yes; 3. Yes; 4. Yes

▶ Check Your Knowledge

Directions: Circle *Yes* if you agree with the statement and *No* if you disagree.

Yes   No   1. Heart attack victims experience the least amount of chest pain when lying down.

Yes   No   2. When taking doctor-prescribed nitroglycerin for chest pain, the person should be sitting or lying down.

Yes   No   3. A stroke victim should have his or her head slightly raised.

Yes   No   4. Most asthma victims will usually have a physician-prescribed inhaler.

Yes   No   5. A victim who is breathing fast (hyperventilating) should be encouraged to breathe slowly by holding inhaled air for several seconds, then exhaling slowly.

Yes   No   6. Splash or sprinkle water on a person who has fainted.

Yes   No   7. Have a fainted victim inhale smelling salts or ammonia inhalants.

Yes   No   8. Place a strong stick or similar object between a seizure victim's teeth.

Yes   No   9. A person having seizures always requires medical care.

Yes   No   10. If in doubt about whether a victim is having an insulin reaction or is in a diabetic coma, give sugar to a responsive victim who can swallow.

Answers: 1. No; 2. Yes; 3. Yes; 4. Yes; 5. Yes; 6. No; 7. No; 8. No; 9. No; 10. Yes

Poisoning

▶ Poisons

A <u>poison</u> (also known as a *toxin*) is any substance that impairs health or causes death by its chemical action when it enters the body or comes in contact with the skin **Figure 13-1** .

▶ Ingested (Swallowed) Poisons

<u>Ingested poisoning</u> occurs when the victim swallows a toxic substance. Fortunately, most poisons ingested have low toxicity or are swallowed in amounts so small that severe poisoning rarely occurs. However, the potential for severe or fatal poisoning is always present.

Recognizing Ingested Poisoning

The signs of ingested poisoning include the following:
- Abdominal pain and cramping
- Nausea or vomiting
- Diarrhea
- Burns, odor, or stains around and in the mouth
- Drowsiness or unconsciousness
- Poison containers nearby

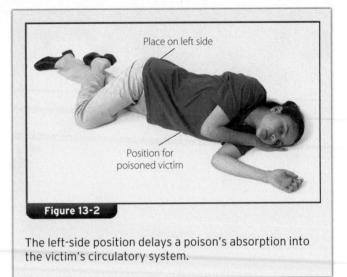

Place on left side

Position for
poisoned victim

Figure 13-2

The left-side position delays a poison's absorption into the victim's circulatory system.

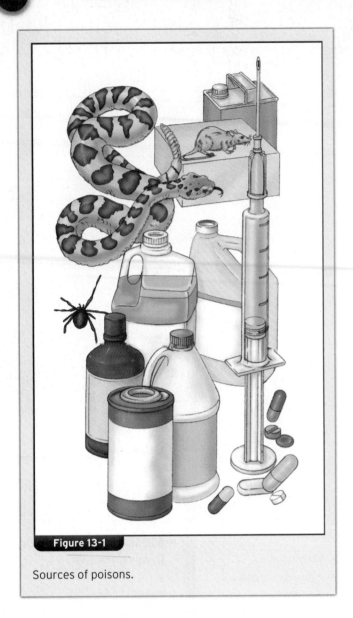

Figure 13-1

Sources of poisons.

Care for Ingested Poisons

To care for victims who have ingested poisons:

1. Determine critical information:
   - Age and size of the victim
   - What was swallowed (read container label; save vomit for analysis.)
   - How much was swallowed (eg, a "taste," half a bottle, a dozen tablets)
   - When it was swallowed
2. If a corrosive or caustic (ie, acid or alkali) substance was swallowed, immediately dilute it by having the victim drink at least one or two 8-ounce glasses of water or milk (cold milk or water tends to absorb heat better than room-temperature or warmer liquids).

3. For a responsive victim, call the poison control center immediately at 1-800-222-1222. Some poisons do not cause harm until hours later, whereas others do damage immediately. More than 75% of poisonings can be treated by following the instructions given over the telephone from the **poison control center**. The center also will advise you if medical care is needed. Poison control centers routinely follow up calls to check whether additional symptoms or unexpected effects are occurring.
4. For an unresponsive victim, check breathing and treat accordingly. Call 9-1-1 or the local emergency number. Monitor breathing often.
5. Place the victim on his or her left side (known as the recovery position). This positions the end of the stomach where it enters the small intestine (pylorus) straight up. In this position, gravity will delay (by as much as 2 hours) the poison's advance into the small intestine, where absorption into the victim's circulatory system is faster **Figure 13-2**. The side position also helps prevent breathing foreign materials into the lungs if vomiting begins. Do not induce vomiting.
6. Give **activated charcoal** if the poison control center advises **Figure 13-3**. Activated charcoal acts like a sponge to bind and keep the poison in the digestive system, thus preventing its absorption into the blood. Although activated charcoal may appear similar to burnt-toast scrapings and charcoal briquettes, these items cannot be used for poisoning.

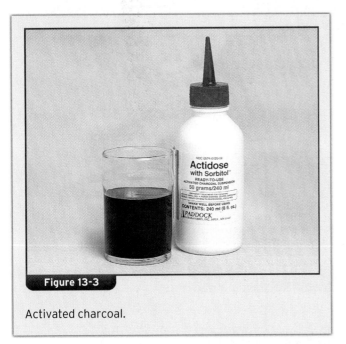

Figure 13-3

Activated charcoal.

Not all chemicals, however, are absorbed well by activated charcoal, including acids and alkalis (eg, bleach, ammonia), potassium, iron, alcohol, methanol, kerosene, cyanide, malathion, and ferrous sulfate.

A drawback of activated charcoal is its grittiness and appearance. Trying to improve the taste or consistency by adding chocolate syrup, sherbet, ice cream, milk, or other flavoring agents only decreases the charcoal's binding capacity. Place the charcoal mixture in an opaque container and have the victim sip it through a straw so it will be more palatable. First aiders should give only the premixed form.

Although activated charcoal is an inexpensive, safe, and effective means for decreasing poison absorption, pharmacies do not routinely stock it. Activated charcoal can be ordered by mail order on the internet.

7. Save poison containers, plants, and the victim's vomit to help medical personnel identify the poison.

> **CAUTION**
>
> DO NOT give water or milk to dilute poisons other than caustic or corrosive substances (acids and alkalis) unless told to do so by staff at a poison center. Fluids may dissolve a dry poison (eg, tablets or capsules) more rapidly and fill up the stomach, forcing stomach contents (ie, the poison) into the small intestine, where poisons are absorbed faster.
>
> DO NOT cause vomiting—there is no evidence that it helps.

▶ Alcohol and Other Drug Emergencies

Poisoning caused by an overdose or abuse of medications and other substances, including alcohol, is common. The most commonly abused drug in the United States is alcohol.

Recognizing Alcohol Intoxication

Helping an intoxicated person is often difficult because the individual may be belligerent and combative. Also, personal hygiene is sometimes less than optimal. However, it is important that alcohol abusers be helped and not just labeled as "drunks." Their condition may be quite serious, even life-threatening. Although the following signs indicate alcohol intoxication, some may also mean illness or injury other than alcohol abuse, such as diabetes or heat injury:

- The odor of alcohol on a person's breath or clothing
- Unsteady, staggering walking
- Slurred speech and the inability to carry on a conversation
- Nausea and vomiting
- Flushed face

> **CAUTION**
>
> DO NOT let an intoxicated person sleep on his or her back.
>
> DO NOT leave an intoxicated person alone.
>
> DO NOT try to handle a hostile intoxicated person by yourself. Find a safe place, then call the police for help.

Care for Alcohol Intoxication

First aid for an intoxicated person includes these steps:

1. Look for injuries. Alcohol can mask pain.
2. Monitor breathing.
3. If the intoxicated person is lying down, place him or her in the recovery position. Rolling the victim onto the left side not only reduces the likelihood of vomiting and aspiration of vomit, but also delays absorption of alcohol into the bloodstream.
4. Call the poison control center (1-800-222-1222) for advice or 9-1-1 for help.
5. Provide emotional support, but if the victim becomes violent, leave the scene, call 9-1-1, and find a safe place until police arrive.

Swallowed Poison

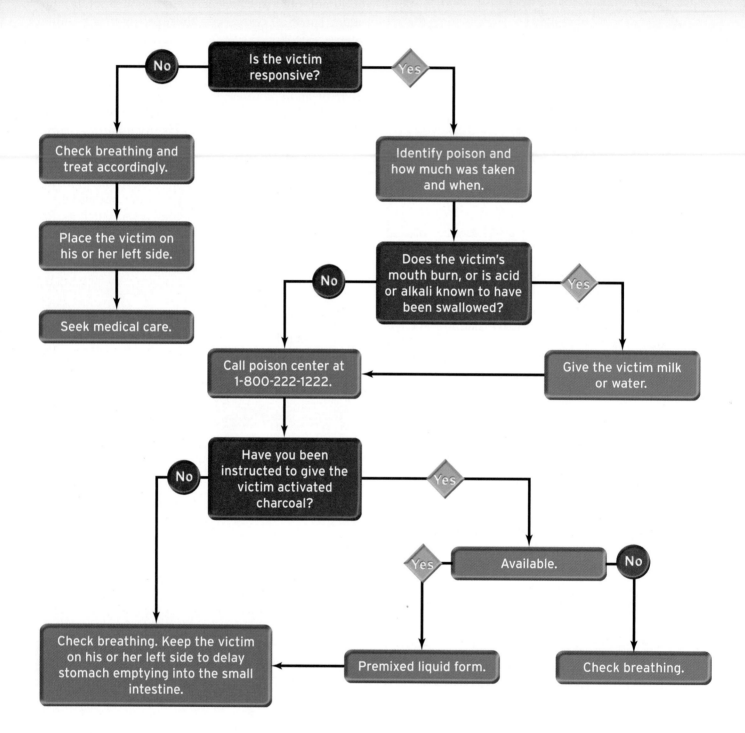

6. If the intoxicated victim has been exposed to the cold, suspect hypothermia and move the person to a warm environment whenever possible. Remove wet clothing and cover the individual with warm blankets. Handle a hypothermic victim gently because rough handling could induce cardiac arrest.

Recognizing Drug Overdose

The condition of a person suffering from drug overdose may be quite serious, even life-threatening. The signs of drug overdose include the following:

- Drowsiness, anxiety, or agitation
- Dilated (large) or constricted (small) pupils
- Confusion
- Hallucinations

Care for a Drug Overdose

Care for a drug overdose is the same as that for alcohol intoxication:

1. Look for injuries. Drugs can mask pain.
2. Monitor breathing.
3. If the victim is lying down, place him or her in the recovery position. Rolling the victim onto the left side not only reduces the likelihood of vomiting and aspiration of vomit, but also delays absorption of drugs into the bloodstream.
4. Call the poison control center (1-800-222-1222) for advice or 9-1-1 for help.
5. Provide emotional support, but if the victim becomes violent, leave the scene, call 9-1-1, and find a safe place until police arrive.
6. If the victim has been exposed to the cold, suspect hypothermia and move the person to a warm environment whenever possible. Remove wet clothing and cover the individual with warm blankets. Handle a hypothermic victim gently because rough handling could induce a cardiac arrest.

▶ Carbon Monoxide Poisoning

Carbon monoxide (CO) victims are often unaware of its presence. The gas is invisible, tasteless, odorless, and non-irritating. It is produced by the incomplete burning of organic material such as gasoline, wood, paper, charcoal, coal, and natural gas. The most common causes of CO poisoning are malfunctioning non-electric heaters and furnaces, and automobiles running in closed spaces. All homes should have a CO detector, and furnaces should be inspected yearly.

Recognizing Carbon Monoxide Poisoning

It is difficult to tell if a person is a CO victim. The signs and symptoms of CO poisoning are as follows:

- Bright red skin
- Headache
- Ringing in the ears (tinnitus)
- Chest pain (angina)
- Muscle weakness
- Nausea and vomiting
- Dizziness and visual changes (blurred or double vision)
- Unresponsiveness
- Breathing has stopped

The following conditions indicate possible CO poisoning:

- The symptoms come and go.
- The symptoms worsen or improve in certain places or at certain times of the day.
- The symptoms can be confused with the flu.
- People around the victim have similar symptoms.
- Pets seem ill.

Care for Carbon Monoxide Poisoning

To care for victims of CO poisoning:

1. Get the victim out of the toxic environment and into fresh air immediately.
2. Call 9-1-1.
3. Monitor breathing.
4. Place an unresponsive victim on the left side (the recovery position).
5. Seek medical care. All suspected CO victims should obtain a blood test to determine the level of CO in the blood.

▶ Plant Poisoning

About 50% of people exposed to poison ivy, poison oak, and poison sumac are allergic to the plant and will react to it. More than 60 plants can cause allergic reactions, but poison ivy, poison oak, and poison sumac are by far the most common Figure 13-4 A-C .

Recognizing Plant Poisoning

An allergic reaction may begin as early as 6 hours after contact, but usually it occurs 24 to 72 hours after exposure. The signs of plant poisoning include the following:

- Rash Figure 13-5
- Itching
- Redness
- Blisters
- Swelling

Care for Plant Poisoning

To care for plant poisoning:

1. Those who know they have been in contact with a poisonous plant should decontaminate the skin as soon as possible (within 5 minutes for

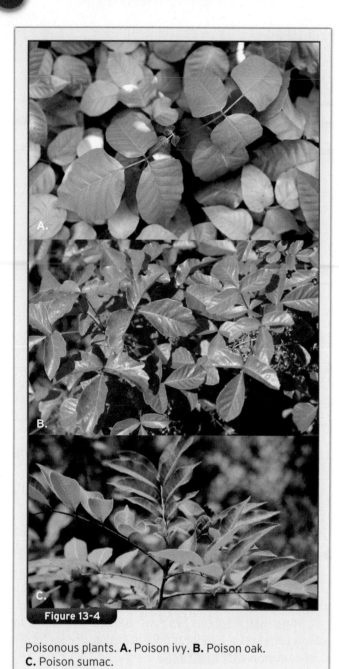

Figure 13-4

Poisonous plants. **A.** Poison ivy. **B.** Poison oak. **C.** Poison sumac.

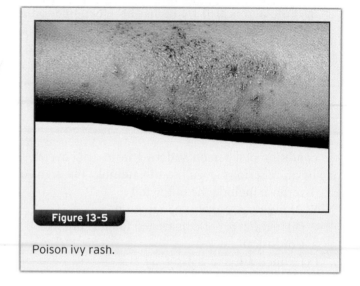

Figure 13-5

Poison ivy rash.

sensitive people, up to 1 hour for moderately sensitive individuals). Use soap and cold water to clean the skin of the oily resin or apply rubbing (isopropyl) alcohol liberally (not in swab-type dabs). If too little isopropyl alcohol is used, the oil will actually spread to another site and enlarge the injury. Rinse with water to remove the solubilized material. Water removes the urushiol (plant resin) from the skin, oxidizes and inactivates it, and does not penetrate the skin, as do solvents. Unfortunately, most victims do not know about their contact until several hours or days later, when the itching and rash begin, which is too late to use the described procedure.

2. If the reaction is mild, the person can soak in a lukewarm bath sprinkled with one to two cups of colloidal oatmeal, such as Aveeno colloidal oatmeal, or apply any of the following:
   - Calamine lotion (calamine ointment if the skin becomes dry and cracked) or zinc oxide
   - Baking soda paste: 1 teaspoon of water mixed with 3 teaspoons of baking soda

3. If the reaction is mild to moderate, care for the skin as you would for a mild reaction and use a physician-prescribed corticosteroid ointment. Oral antihistamines such as Benadryl often are used in conjunction with prescription ointment or cream to help decrease itching.

4. For a severe reaction, follow the same care guidelines for the skin and use a physician-prescribed oral corticosteroid (eg, prednisone). Apply a topical corticosteroid ointment or cream.

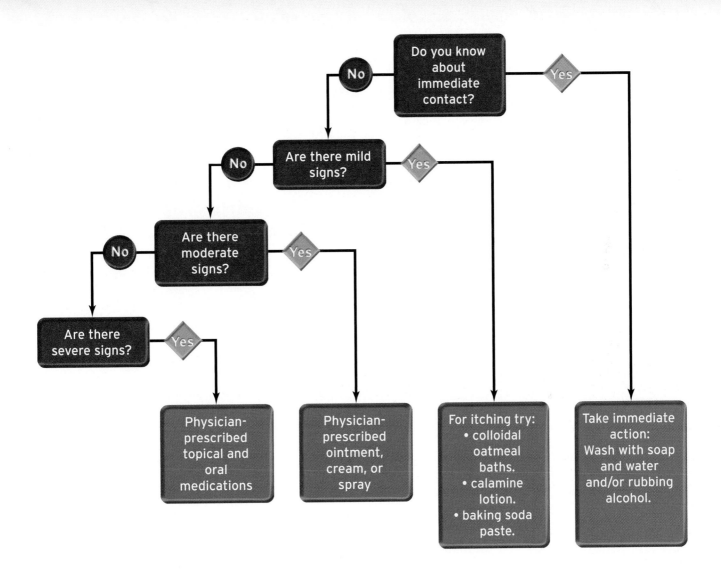

▶ Poisoning

What to Look For | What to Do

Ingested (swallowed) poisoning
- Abdominal pain and cramping
- Nausea or vomiting
- Diarrhea
- Burns, odor, or stains around and in mouth
- Drowsiness or unresponsiveness
- Poison container nearby

1. Determine the age and size of the victim, what and how much was swallowed, and when it was swallowed.
2. If victim is responsive, call the poison control center at 1-800-222-1222. If advised, give activated charcoal. The center will advise if medical care is needed.
3. If victim is unresponsive, open airway, check breathing, and treat accordingly. If breathing, place on left side in recovery position. Call 9-1-1.

Alcohol intoxication
- Alcohol odor on breath or clothing
- Unsteadiness, staggering
- Confusion
- Slurred speech
- Nausea and vomiting
- Flushed face

1. If the victim is responsive:
   - Monitor breathing.
   - Look for injuries.
   - Place in recovery position.
   - Call poison control center for advice (1-800-222-1222).
   - If victim becomes violent, leave area and call 9-1-1.
2. If victim is unresponsive, open airway, check breathing, and treat accordingly.

Drug overdose
- Drowsiness, agitation, anxiety, hyperactivity
- Change in pupil size
- Confusion
- Hallucinations

1. If the victim is responsive:
   - Monitor breathing.
   - Look for injuries.
   - Place in recovery position.
   - Call poison control center for advice (1-800-222-1222).
   - If victim becomes violent, leave area and call 9-1-1.
2. If victim is unresponsive, open airway, check breathing, and treat accordingly.

Carbon monoxide poisoning
- Headache
- Ringing in ears
- Chest pain
- Muscle weakness
- Nausea and vomiting
- Dizziness and vision difficulties
- Unresponsiveness
- Breathing and heart stopped
- Bright red skin

1. Move victim to fresh air.
2. Call 9-1-1.
3. Monitor breathing.
4. Place unresponsive breathing victim in recovery position.

Plant (contact) poisoning
- Rash
- Itching
- Redness
- Blisters
- Swelling

1. For known contact, immediately wash with soap and water.
2. For mild reaction, use one or more:
   - 1–2 cups of colloidal oatmeal in bathwater
   - Calamine lotion
   - Baking soda paste
3. For severe reactions, perform step 2 and seek medical care.

▶ Ready for Review

- A poison is any substance that impairs health or causes death by its chemical action when it enters the body or comes in contact with the skin.
- Ingested poison occurs when the victim swallows a toxic substance.
- For a responsive poisoned victim, call the poison control center at 1-800-222-1222. For an unresponsive poisoned victim, call 9-1-1 and check for breathing.
- Do not induce vomiting in a poisoned victim.
- Do not use activated charcoal unless instructed to do so by a poison control center.
- If a corrosive or caustic (ie acid or alkali) substance was swallowed, dilute with water or milk.
- If an intoxicated person or a person using drugs becomes violent, leave the scene, call 9-1-1, and find a safe place until the police arrive.
- Carbon monoxide is a gas that is invisible, tasteless, odorless, and nonirritating. It is difficult to tell if a person is a CO victim.
- Mild contacting of poison plants may be treated using calamine lotion or baking soda paste. For severe reactions, a physician-prescribed medication may be necessary.

▶ Vital Vocabulary

__activated charcoal__ Powdered charcoal that has been treated to increase its powers of absorption. Used to treat patients who have ingested poisons.

__carbon monoxide (CO)__ A colorless, odorless, poisonous gas formed by incomplete combustion, such as in fire.

__ingested poisoning__ Poisoning caused by swallowing a toxic substance.

__poison__ Any substance that impairs health or causes death by its chemical action when it enters the body or comes in contact with the skin; also known as a _toxin_.

__poison control center__ Medical facility providing immediate, free, expert advice anytime by calling 1-800-222-1222.

▶ Assessment in Action

A 24-year-old driver is waiting in his truck until workers can load it. He's left the motor running to keep the heater on and has closed all the windows and doors because of the subfreezing outside temperatures. After 30 minutes, when the workers come to tell him they're ready, he is slumped unresponsive over the wheel.

prep kit

Directions: Circle _Yes_ if you agree with the statement and _No_ if you disagree.

Yes No 1. One of the first things to do is check for breathing.

Yes No 2. You suspect poisoning by carbon monoxide because of the running truck engine.

Yes No 3. Call the poison control center at 1-800-222-1222.

Yes No 4. Give this victim activated charcoal.

Answers: **1.** Yes; **2.** Yes; **3.** No; **4.** No

▶ Check Your Knowledge

Directions: Circle _Yes_ if you agree with the statement and _No_ if you disagree.

Yes No 1. If a corrosive or caustic substance was swallowed, you may dilute it by having the victim drink water or milk.

Yes No 2. For a responsive poisoned victim, call a poison control center immediately.

Yes No 3. Use activated charcoal for an ingested poisoned victim if advised by poison control.

Yes No 4. Place a swallowed poison victim on his or her left side to delay the poison from going into the small intestine.

Yes No 5. Place an intoxicated person who is asleep on his or her back.

Yes No 6. If an intoxicated or drugged person becomes violent, leave the scene and let law enforcement officers handle the situation.

Yes No 7. You can detect carbon monoxide by its unique smell.

Yes No 8. Calamine lotion can help relieve itching caused by poison ivy, oak, or sumac.

Yes No 9. Some cases of poison ivy, oak, or sumac require medical care.

Yes No 10. Causing an ingested poisoned victim to vomit is a recommended first aid procedure.

Answers: **1.** Yes; **2.** Yes; **3.** Yes; **4.** Yes; **5.** No; **6.** Yes; **7.** No; **8.** Yes; **9.** Yes; **10.** No

Bites and Stings

▶ Animal and Human Bites

It is estimated that one of every two Americans will be bitten at some time by an animal or by another person. As it is commonly interpreted, in this section the term *animal bite* refers to a bite by a mammal, not an insect or a reptile. Dogs are responsible for about 80% of all animal bite injuries **Figure 14-1**. Animal bites represent a major, largely unrecognized public health problem. See **Table 14-1** for the average number of animal-related deaths in the United States each year.

Rabies

Rabies is caused by a virus found in warm-blooded animals. The disease spreads from one animal to another through saliva, usually through a bite or by licking.

An animal should be considered possibly rabid if:

- The animal attacked without provocation.
- The animal acted strangely, that is, out of character (eg, a usually friendly dog is aggressive or a wild fox seems docile and "friendly").
- The animal was a high-risk species (skunk, raccoon, or bat).

Recognizing an Animal Bite

An animal bite has the following characteristics:

- A puncture wound from an animal's sharp, pointed teeth.
- Tissue and skin can be crushed.
- Open wound on fingers, knuckles and/or hand.
- Animal might be present.

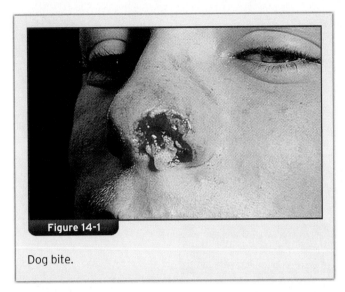

Figure 14-1

Dog bite.

Table 14-1	Animal-Related Human Deaths in the United States (1991-2001)

Animal	Average number of deaths each year
Venomous animals	
Snake	5.2
Spider	6
Scorpion	0.45
Hornet, bee, wasp	48.5
Centipede	0.45
Other specified venomous arthropod	6
Venomous marine animal	0.18
Other specified venomous animal	2.1
Total venomous	68.88
Nonvenomous animals	
Dog	18.9
Rat	0.27
Nonvenomous snake	0
Other animals except arthropod	4
Other specified animal*	76.9
Unspecified animal	4
Total nonvenomous	104.07
Overall total	172.95

*Note that this category includes bitten or struck by other mammals, contact with marine animal, bitten or stung by nonvenomous insect or other nonvenomous arthropods, bitten or struck by crocodile or alligator, bitten or confronted by other reptiles.
Source: Adapted from Langley RL: Animal-related fatalities in the United States: An update. *Wilderness Environ Med* 16(2):67-74.

Care for an Animal Bite

To care for an animal bite:

1. If the victim was bitten in the United States (except for the area along the border with Mexico) by a healthy domestic dog or cat, the animal will likely be confined and observed for 10 days for any illness. If necessary, a veterinarian will kill the animal (domesticated or wild), decapitate it, and send the head to a laboratory for analysis. If the animal is dead when you find it, transport the entire body; do not attempt decapitation (precautions must be taken to prevent exposure to potentially infected tissues and saliva).

    Report animal bites to the police or animal control officers; they should be the ones to capture the animal for observation. If the dog or cat escapes and is not suspected to be rabid, consult local public health officials.

    If the victim was bitten in the United States by a skunk, raccoon, bat, fox, or other mammal, it should be considered a rabies exposure, and treatment should be started *immediately*. The only exception is when the bite occurred in a part of the continental United States known to be free of rabies. If the wild animal is captured, it should be killed and its head shipped to a qualified laboratory immediately.

2. If the wound is not bleeding heavily, wash with soap and water. Avoid scrubbing, which can bruise the tissues.

3. Flush the wound thoroughly with running water under pressure.

4. Control bleeding with direct pressure.

5. Cover the wound with a sterile or clean dressing. Do *not* close the wound with tape or butterfly bandages, which traps bacteria in the wound and increases the chance of infection.

6. Seek medical care for further wound cleaning and a possible tetanus shot. The physician will determine if sutures are needed to close the wound. If needed, a vaccination series against rabies will be started.

Care for a Human Bite

The human mouth contains a wide range of bacteria, so the chance of infection is greater from a human bite than from the bites of other warm-blooded animals.

To care for a human bite:

1. If the wound is not bleeding heavily, wash it with soap and water. Avoid scrubbing, which can bruise tissues.

Animal Bites

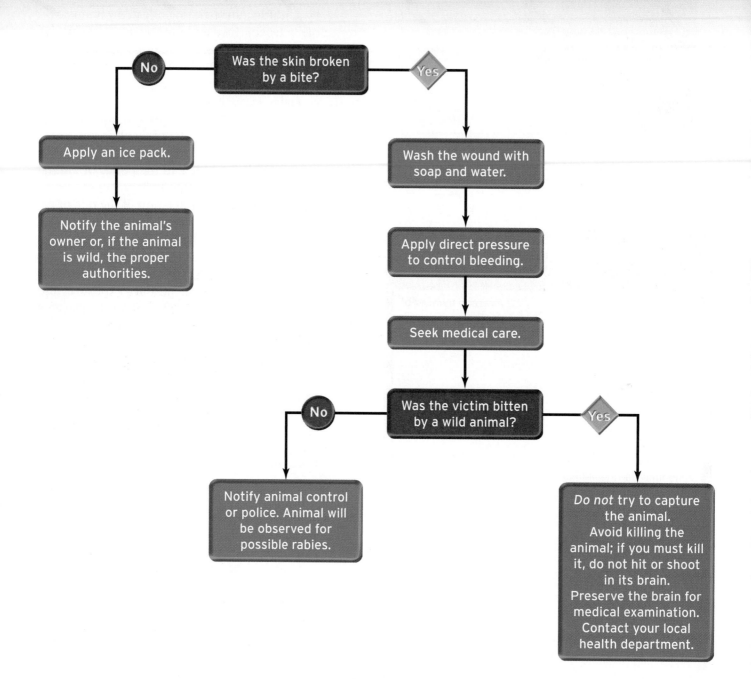

Was the skin broken by a bite?

No → Apply an ice pack. → Notify the animal's owner or, if the animal is wild, the proper authorities.

Yes → Wash the wound with soap and water. → Apply direct pressure to control bleeding. → Seek medical care. →

Was the victim bitten by a wild animal?

No → Notify animal control or police. Animal will be observed for possible rabies.

Yes → *Do not* try to capture the animal. Avoid killing the animal; if you must kill it, do not hit or shoot in its brain. Preserve the brain for medical examination. Contact your local health department.

2. Flush the wound thoroughly with running water under pressure.
3. Control bleeding with direct pressure.
4. Cover the wound with a sterile or clean dressing.
5. Seek medical care for possible further wound cleaning, a tetanus shot, and sutures to close the wound (if needed).

CAUTION

DO NOT close a bite wound with tape or butterfly bandages. Closing the wound traps bacteria in the wound, increasing the chance of infection.

▶ Snakebites

Each year in the United States, 40,000 to 50,000 people are bitten by snakes, 7,000 to 8,000 of them by venomous snakes **Figure 14-2**. Only four snake species in the United States are venomous: rattlesnakes **Figure 14-3** (which account for about 65% of all venomous snakebites and nearly all the snakebite deaths in the United States), copperheads **Figure 14-4**, water moccasins **Figure 14-5** (also known as cottonmouths), and coral snakes **Figure 14-6**.

Rattlesnakes, copperheads, and water moccasins are all pit vipers. Pit vipers have three common characteristics:

- Triangular, flat heads wider than their necks
- Elliptical pupils (cat's eyes)
- Heat-sensitive pit between the eye and the nostril on each side of the head

The coral snake is small and colorful, with a black snout and a series of bright red, yellow, and black bands around its body (every other band is yellow). At least one species of venomous snakes is found in every state except Alaska, Maine, and Hawaii **Figure 14-7**. Venomous snakes from other countries also pose a snakebite problem.

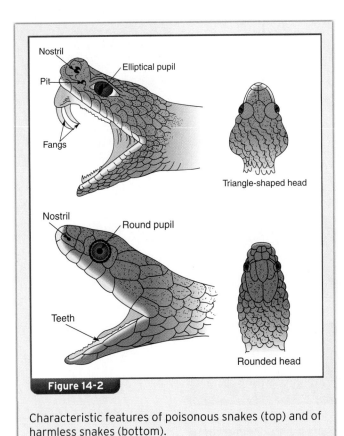

Figure 14-2

Characteristic features of poisonous snakes (top) and of harmless snakes (bottom).

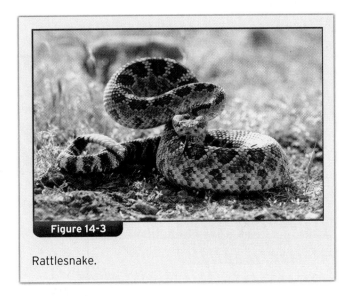

Figure 14-3

Rattlesnake.

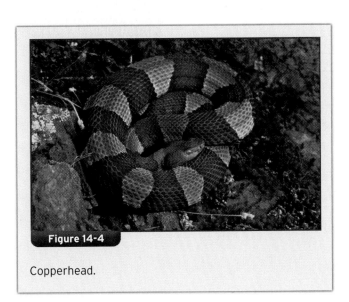

Figure 14-4

Copperhead.

Snakebites

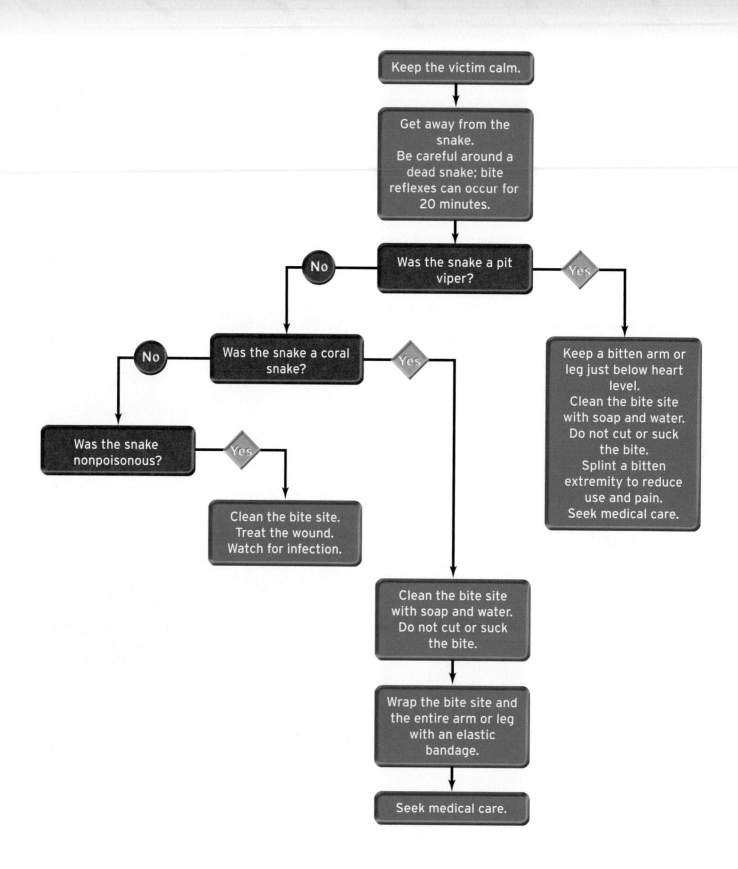

Keep the victim calm.

Get away from the snake.
Be careful around a dead snake; bite reflexes can occur for 20 minutes.

Was the snake a pit viper?

No

Yes

Was the snake a coral snake?

No

Yes

Keep a bitten arm or leg just below heart level.
Clean the bite site with soap and water.
Do not cut or suck the bite.
Splint a bitten extremity to reduce use and pain.
Seek medical care.

Was the snake nonpoisonous?

Yes

Clean the bite site.
Treat the wound.
Watch for infection.

Clean the bite site with soap and water.
Do not cut or suck the bite.

Wrap the bite site and the entire arm or leg with an elastic bandage.

Seek medical care.

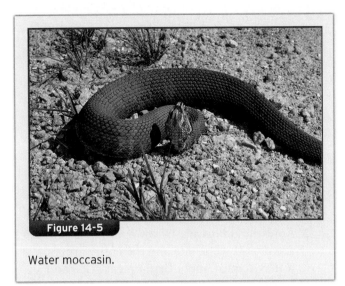

Figure 14-5

Water moccasin.

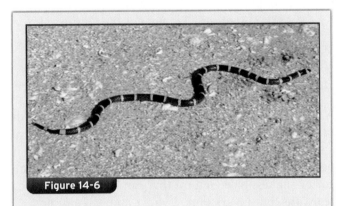

Figure 14-6

Coral snake; the United States' most venomous snake.

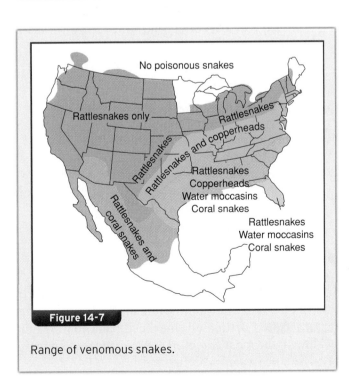

Figure 14-7

Range of venomous snakes.

Recognizing a Pit Viper Bite

The signs of a pit viper bite include the following:

- Severe burning pain at the bite site
- Two small puncture wounds about one-half inch apart (some cases may have only one fang mark) **Figure 14-8**
- Swelling (happens within 5 minutes and can involve an entire extremity)
- Discoloration and blood-filled blisters, possibly developing in 6 to 10 hours **Figure 14-9**
- In severe cases, nausea, vomiting, sweating, and weakness

FYI

Dry Snake Bites

In about 25% of poisonous snakebites, there is no venom injection, only fang and tooth wounds (known as a "dry" bite).

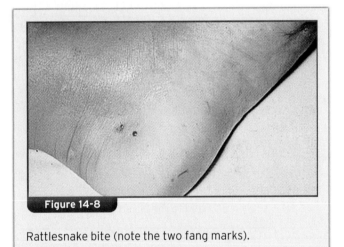

Figure 14-8

Rattlesnake bite (note the two fang marks).

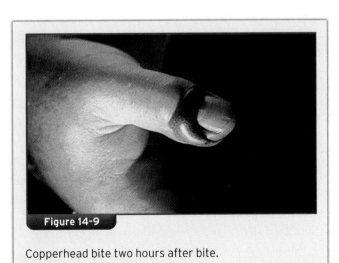

Figure 14-9

Copperhead bite two hours after bite.

Care for a Pit Viper Bite

The Wilderness Medical Society lists the following guidelines for dealing with bites by pit vipers:

1. Get the victim and bystanders away from the snake. Snakes have been known to bite more than once. Pit vipers can strike about one half of their body length. Be careful around a decapitated snake head—bite reflexes can persist for 20 minutes or more.

2. Do not attempt to capture or kill the snake. It wastes valuable time, there is a risk of additional bites, and identification of the snake is not usually needed, because the same antivenin is used for all pit viper bites.

3. Keep the victim calm and limit movement. If possible, carry the victim or have the victim walk very slowly to help minimize exertion.

4. Gently wash the bitten area with soap and water. Any ring(s) or jewelry that might reduce blood circulation if swelling occurs should be removed.

5. Stabilize the bitten extremity (arm or leg) with a sling or a splint as you would for a fracture. Keep the extremity below heart level despite the fact that swelling may occur.

6. Seek medical care *immediately*. This is the most important thing to do for the victim. Antivenin must be given within four hours of the bite (not every venomous snakebite requires antivenin).

CAUTION

DO NOT cut the victim's skin.
DO NOT attempt to suck out the venom.
DO NOT apply ice or cold to the bitten area.

FYI

Antivenin
Identifying the type of pit viper is not very important because the same <u>antivenin</u> is used to counteract all North American pit viper venom.

Recognizing a Coral Snake Bite

The coral snake is America's most venomous snake, but it rarely bites people. The coral snake has short fangs and tends to hang on and "chew" its venom into the victim rather than strike and release, like a pit viper.

Symptoms might include:
- Minimal pain
- Sagging or drooping of upper eyelids
- Weakness
- Pricking, tingling of skin (often numb at bite site)
- Double vision (seeing two of a single object)
- Difficulty in swallowing
- Sweating
- Abnormal flow of saliva

Care for a Coral Snake Bite

To care for a coral snake bite:

1. Keep the victim calm and limit movement.
2. Gently clean the bite site with soap and water.
3. Apply mild pressure by wrapping an elastic bandage over the bite site and the entire arm or leg—it may require more than one elastic bandage to cover the entire arm or leg. You should apply pressure only if the bite is from a coral snake, not any of the pit vipers. Do *not* cut the victim's skin or use any suction device.
4. Seek medical care for antivenin.

Recognizing a Nonpoisonous Snakebite

A nonpoisonous snake leaves a horseshoe shape of toothmarks on the victim's skin. If you are not positive about a snake, assume it was venomous. Some so-called nonpoisonous North American snakes, such as hognose and garter snakes, have venom that can cause painful local reactions, but no systemic (whole-body) symptoms.

A nonpoisonous snakebite results in:
- Feeling of a mild to moderate pinch
- Curved lines (horseshoe shaped) of tiny pinpricks on the skin that correspond with the rows of sharp, pointy teeth
- Bleeding
- Mild itching

Care for a Nonpoisonous Snake Bite

To care for a nonpoisonous snakebite:

1. Gently clean the bite site with soap and water.
2. Care for the bite as you would a minor wound—apply antibiotic ointment and cover the bite site with a sterile or clean dressing.
3. Seek medical advice.

▶ Insect Stings

Severe allergic reactions to insect stings are reported by less than 1% of the population in the United States **Figure 14-10** . Fortunately, localized pain, itching, and swelling—the most common consequences of an insect bite—can be treated with first aid.

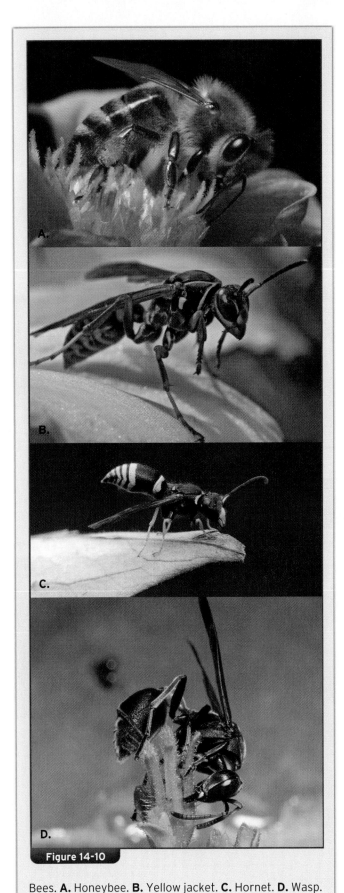

Figure 14-10

Bees. **A.** Honeybee. **B.** Yellow jacket. **C.** Hornet. **D.** Wasp.

Recognizing an Insect Sting

A rule of thumb is that the sooner symptoms develop after a sting, the more serious the reaction will be. Common signs of an insect sting are as follows:

- Pain
- Itching
- Swelling

Signs of a severe allergic reaction (anaphylaxis) include the following:

- Difficulty breathing
- Tightness in the chest
- Itchy, burning skin with a rash or hives
- Swelling of the tongue, mouth, or throat
- Dizziness and nausea

Care for an Insect Sting

Most people who have been stung can be treated on site, and everyone should know what to do if a life-threatening allergic reaction (anaphylaxis) occurs. In particular, those who have had a severe reaction to an insect sting should be instructed on what they can do to protect themselves. They also should be advised to wear a medical-alert identification tag stating they are insect allergic.

To care for an insect sting:

1. Check the sting site to see if a stinger and venom sac are embedded in the skin. Bees are the only stinging insects that leave their stingers and venom sacs behind. If the stinger is still embedded, remove it or it will continue to inject poison for 2 or 3 minutes. Do not use tweezers to remove a stinger since this may squeeze more venom into the victim. Scrape the stinger and venom sac away with a hard object such as a long fingernail, credit card, scissor edge, or knife blade **Figure 14-11** .

2. Wash the sting site with soap and water to prevent infection.

3. Apply an ice pack over the sting site to slow absorption of the venom and relieve pain. Because bee venom is acidic, a paste made of baking soda and water can help. Sodium bicarbonate is an alkalinizing agent that draws out fluid and reduces itching and swelling. Wasp venom, however, is alkaline, so apply vinegar or lemon juice.

4. To further relieve pain and itching, some type of pain medication usually is adequate. A topical corticosteroid cream, such as hydrocortisone, can help combat local swelling and itching. An antihistamine may prevent some local symptoms and later reactions if given early, but it works too slowly to counteract a life-threatening allergic reaction.

Insect Stings

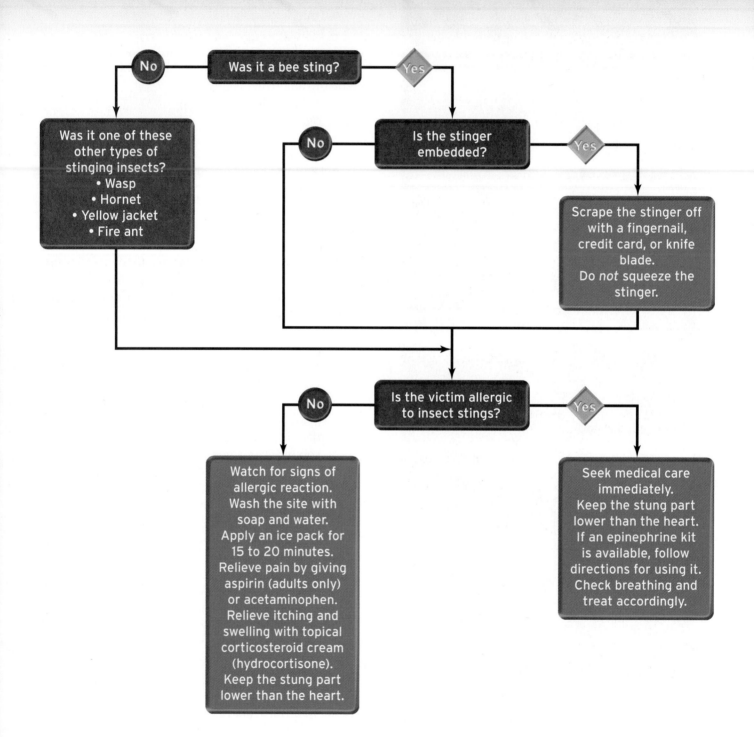

Was it a bee sting?

No

Yes

Was it one of these other types of stinging insects?
- Wasp
- Hornet
- Yellow jacket
- Fire ant

Is the stinger embedded?

No

Yes

Scrape the stinger off with a fingernail, credit card, or knife blade.
Do *not* squeeze the stinger.

Is the victim allergic to insect stings?

No

Yes

Watch for signs of allergic reaction.
Wash the site with soap and water.
Apply an ice pack for 15 to 20 minutes.
Relieve pain by giving aspirin (adults only) or acetaminophen.
Relieve itching and swelling with topical corticosteroid cream (hydrocortisone).
Keep the stung part lower than the heart.

Seek medical care immediately.
Keep the stung part lower than the heart.
If an epinephrine kit is available, follow directions for using it.
Check breathing and treat accordingly.

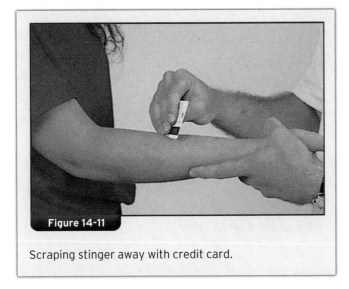

Figure 14-11

Scraping stinger away with credit card.

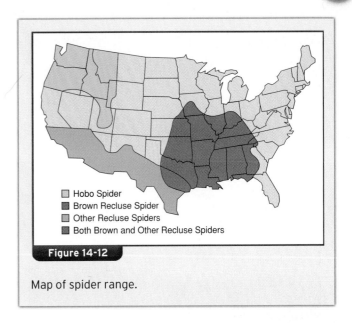

Figure 14-12

Map of spider range.

Hobo Spider
Brown Recluse Spider
Other Recluse Spiders
Both Brown and Other Recluse Spiders

5. Observe the victim for at least 30 minutes for signs of an allergic reaction. Epinephrine is an effective treatment for a person with a severe allergic reaction. A person with a known allergy to insect stings should have a physician-prescribed emergency kit that includes a prefilled auto-injector of epinephrine. Help the victim use it. Because epinephrine is short acting, watch the victim closely for signs of returning anaphylaxis. Inject another dose of epinephrine as often as every 15 minutes, if needed, available, and consistent with the directions for use in the kit. Take the victim to the hospital for additional evaluation.

▶ Spider Bites

Most spiders are venomous, which is how they paralyze and kill their prey. However, most spiders lack an effective delivery system (long fangs and strong jaws) to bite a human. About 60 species of spiders in North America are capable of biting humans, although only a few species have produced significant poisonings **Figure 14-12**. Death occurs rarely and only from bites by brown recluse and black widow spiders.

A spider bite is difficult to diagnose, especially when the spider was not seen or recovered, because the bites typically cause little immediate pain.

Recognizing a Black Widow Spider Bite

Black widow spiders have round abdomens that vary in color from gray to brown to black, depending on the species **Figure 14-13**. In the female black widow, the abdomen is shiny black with a red or yellow spot (often in the shape of an hourglass) or white spots or bands. Black widow spiders are found throughout the world.

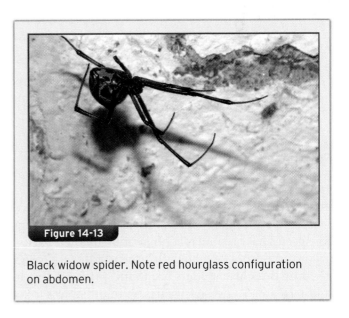

Figure 14-13

Black widow spider. Note red hourglass configuration on abdomen.

Signs of a black widow spider bite can include the following:

- The victim may feel a sharp pinprick when the spider bites, but some victims are not even aware of the bite. Within 15 minutes, a dull, numbing pain develops in the bite area.
- Two small fang marks might be seen as tiny red spots.
- Within 15 minutes to 4 hours, muscle stiffness and cramps occur, usually affecting the abdomen when the bite is on a lower part of the body and the shoulders, back, or chest when the bite is on an upper part. Victims often describe the pain as the most severe they have ever experienced.

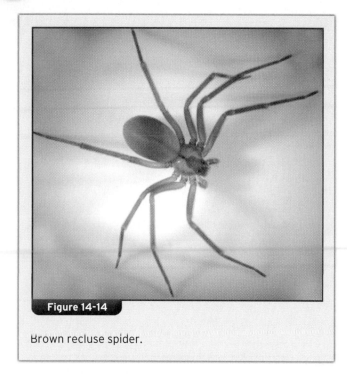

Figure 14-14

Brown recluse spider.

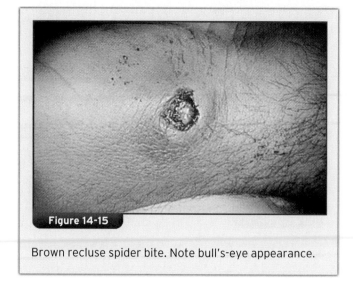

Figure 14-15

Brown recluse spider bite. Note bull's-eye appearance.

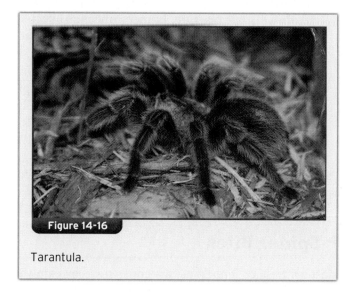

Figure 14-16

Tarantula.

• Headache, chills, fever, heavy sweating, dizziness, nausea, and vomiting appear next. Severe pain around the bite site peaks in 2 to 3 hours and can last 12 to 48 hours.

Recognizing a Brown Recluse Spider Bite

Brown recluse spiders are also known in North America as fiddle-back or violin spiders **Figure 14-14** . They have a violin-shaped figure on their backs (several other spider species have a similar configuration on their backs). Color varies from fawn to dark brown, with darker legs.

Brown recluse spiders are found primarily in the southern and Midwestern states, with other, less toxic, related spiders throughout the rest of the country. They are absent from the Pacific Northwest, where the aggressive house spider, also known as the hobo spider, is found and causes injuries similar to those of the brown recluse.

Signs of a brown recluse and hobo spider bite include the following:

• A local reaction usually occurs within 2 to 8 hours with mild to severe pain at the bite site and redness, swelling, and local itching.

• In 48 to 72 hours, a blister develops at the bite site, becomes red, and bursts. During the early stages, the affected area often takes on a bull's-eye appearance, with a central white area surrounded by a reddened area, ringed by a whitish or blue border **Figure 14-15** . A small, red crater remains, over which a scab forms. When that scab falls away in

a few days, a larger crater remains. That also scabs over and falls off, leaving a yet larger crater. The craters are known as *volcano lesions*. This process of slow tissue destruction can continue for weeks or even months. The ulcer sometimes requires skin grafting.

• Fever, weakness, vomiting, joint pain, and a rash may occur.

• Stomach cramps, nausea, and vomiting may occur.

Recognizing a Tarantula Spider Bite

Tarantulas bite only when vigorously provoked or roughly handled **Figure 14-16** . The bite varies from almost painless to a deep throbbing pain lasting up to 1 hour. The tarantula, when upset, will roughly scratch the lower surface of its abdomen with its legs and flick hairs onto the

Spider Bites and Scorpion Stings

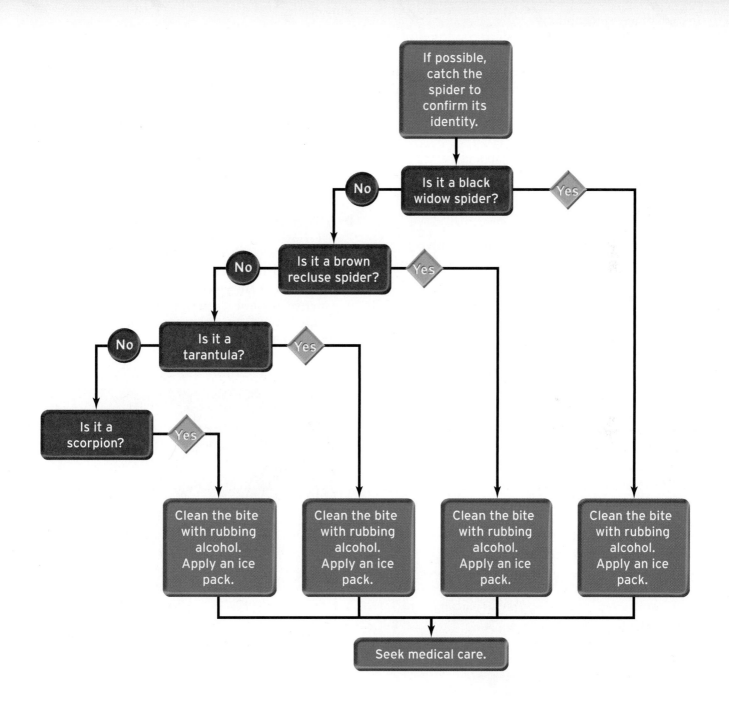

invader's skin. The hairs cause itching and hives that can last several weeks. Treatment is hydrocortisone cream, antihistamines, and a pain medication.

Care for All Spider Bites

To care for any spider bite:
1. If possible, catch the spider to confirm its identity. Even if the body has been crushed, save it for identification (although most spider-bite victims never see the spider). The species helps determine the treatment, so the dead spider (if it can be found) should be taken with the victim to the hospital.
2. Clean the bite area with soap and water or rubbing alcohol.
3. Place an ice pack over the bite to relieve pain and delay the effects of the venom.
4. Monitor breathing.
5. Seek medical care immediately. An antivenin exists for black widow spider bites. It is usually reserved for children (under 6 years), the elderly (over 60 and with high blood pressure), pregnant women, and victims with severe reactions. The antivenin will give relief within 1 to 3 hours. Antivenin for brown recluse and other spider bites is not currently available.

▶ Scorpion Stings

Scorpions look like miniature lobsters, with lobster-like pincers and a long up-curved "tail" with a poisonous stinger **Figure 14-17**. Several species of scorpions inhabit the southwestern United States, but only the bark scorpion poses a threat to humans.

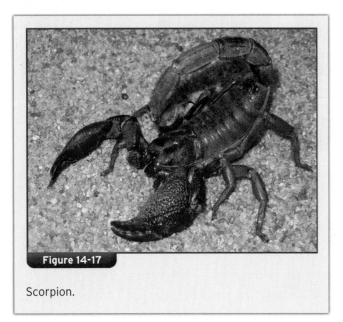

Figure 14-17

Scorpion.

Recognizing a Scorpion Sting

The most frequent symptom of a scorpion sting, especially in an adult victim, is local, immediate pain and burning around the sting site. Later, numbness or tingling occurs.

Care for a Scorpion Sting

To care for a scorpion sting:
1. Monitor breathing.
2. Gently clean the sting site with soap and water or rubbing alcohol.
3. Apply an ice pack over the sting site.
4. Seek medical care. Small children are prime candidates for receiving antivenin. An antivenin is available only in Arizona.

▶ Tick Bites

Most tick bites are harmless, although ticks can carry serious diseases. If a tick is carrying a disease, the longer it stays embedded, the greater the chance of disease being transmitted. Because its bite is painless, a tick can remain embedded for days without the victim realizing it **Figure 14-18 A, B**.

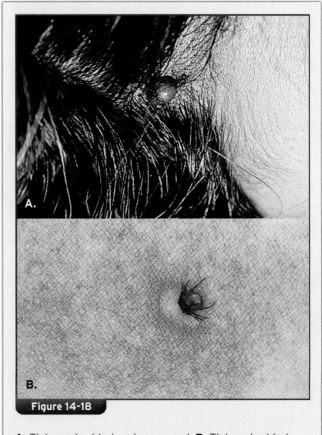

Figure 14-18

A. Ticks embedded and engorged. **B.** Tick embedded.

Care for Tick Bites

To care for tick bites:

1. To remove an embedded tick, use tweezers or one of the specialized tick-removal tools **Figure 14-19**. Grasp the tick as close to the skin as possible and lift the tick with enough force to "tent" the skin surface. Hold in this position until the tick lets go. This may take several seconds. Do not pull hard enough to break the tick apart, because this will leave parts of the tick behind that will cause infection.

2. After the tick has been removed, wash the bite site with soap and water. Apply rubbing alcohol to further disinfect the area.

3. Apply an ice pack to reduce pain.

4. Apply calamine lotion to relieve any itching. Keep the area clean.

5. Watch the bite site for 1 month for a rash. If a rash appears, seek medical care. Watch for other signs, such as fever, muscle or joint aches, sensitivity to bright light, and paralysis that begins with leg weakness.

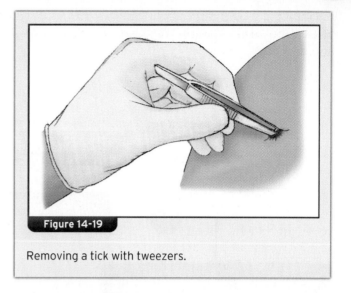

Figure 14-19

Removing a tick with tweezers.

CAUTION

DO NOT use the following methods to remove a tick:

- Petroleum jelly
- Fingernail polish
- Gasoline or rubbing alcohol
- Blown-out hot match

Tick Removal

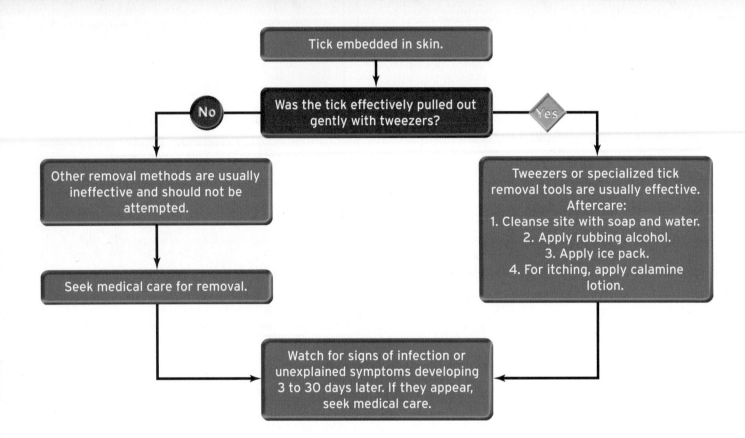

Tick embedded in skin.

Was the tick effectively pulled out gently with tweezers?

No

Yes

Other removal methods are usually ineffective and should not be attempted.

Seek medical care for removal.

Tweezers or specialized tick removal tools are usually effective.
Aftercare:
1. Cleanse site with soap and water.
2. Apply rubbing alcohol.
3. Apply ice pack.
4. For itching, apply calamine lotion.

Watch for signs of infection or unexplained symptoms developing 3 to 30 days later. If they appear, seek medical care.

▶ Bites and Stings

What to Look For	What to Do
Animal and human bites • Torn tissue • Bleeding	1. Wash wound with soap and water under pressure. 2. Flush wound thoroughly. 3. Control bleeding. 4. Seek medical care.
Poisonous snake bites • Severe, burning pain • Small puncture wounds • Swelling • Nausea, vomiting, sweating, weakness • Discoloration and blood-filled blisters developing hours after the bite	1. Get away from the snake. 2. Limit victim's movement and keep bitten extremity below heart level. 3. Call 9-1-1. 4. Gently wash area with soap and water. 5. For a coral snake bite, apply mild pressure by wrapping the entire affected arm or leg with an elastic bandage.
Insect stings • Pain • Itching • Swelling • Severe allergic reaction, including breathing problems	1. Scrape away any stinger. 2. Wash with soap and water. 3. Apply an ice or cold pack. 4. Give pain medication, hydrocortisone cream, and an antihistamine. 5. Observe for at least 30 minutes for signs of severe allergic reaction. Call 9-1-1 if a severe allergic reaction occurs. If victim has an epinephrine auto-injector, help victim use it.

Spider bites
• Black widow
  • May feel sharp pain
  • Two small fang marks
  • Severe abdominal pain
  • Headache, chills, fever, sweating, dizziness, nausea
• Brown recluse and hobo
  • Blister developing several days later
  • Ulcer in skin
  • Headache, fever, weakness, nausea
	1. Catch spider for identification.
	2. Wash bitten area with soap and water.
	3. Apply an ice or cold pack.
	4. Seek medical care.

Scorpion stings • Pain and burning at sting site • Later, numbness or tingling	1. Wash sting site with soap and water. 2. Apply an ice or cold pack. 3. Seek medical care.
Tick bites • Tick still attached • Rash (especially one shaped like a bull's-eye) • Fever, joint aches, weakness	1. Remove tick. 2. Wash bitten area with soap and water. 3. Apply rubbing alcohol. 4. Apply an ice or cold pack. 5. Watch bitten area for 1 month for rash. Seek medical care if rash or other signs such as fever or muscle joint aches appear.

prep kit

▶ Ready for Review

- Almost half of all Americans will suffer a bite from either an animal or human during their lifetime.
- Flushing animal and human bites with water under pressure is essential to prevent infection.
- Of the poisonous snakes in the United States, pit vipers account for most of the bites.
- Seeking medical care for snakebites is the best first aid procedure. Do not apply ice; do not use suction.
- The sooner symptoms develop after an insect sting, the more serious the reaction will be.
- Only bees leave a stinger in the victim's skin, which should be scraped out.
- Insect stings are usually only a nuisance and painful, but about 1 in every 200 people is dangerously allergic to their venom. Always check and monitor for anaphylaxis. This condition is best treated by injecting epinephrine, which a victim should have with them if they know they are allergic.
- Spiders that bite are seldom seen by the victim.
- Black widows are the most dangerous spider in the United States.
- Seek medical care for all suspected spider bites. Although all spiders are poisonous, most are not capable of biting a human due to short or weak fangs.
- Ticks can carry dangerous diseases. The longer one stays embedded in the skin, the more likely, if it has a disease, of transmitting it to a victim.
- Ticks can successfully be removed using tweezers or a special tick-removal device.

▶ Vital Vocabulary

<u>antivenin</u> An antiserum containing antibodies against reptile or insect venom.

<u>rabies</u> An acute viral infection of the central nervous system transmitted by the bite of an infected animal.

▶ Assessment in Action

A mail carrier is heard crying for help while being attacked by a neighbor's large dog. The dog's owner calls off the dog and takes it inside his house. You run up the street and help the victim over to a nearby yard. You find several severe bite marks on the mail carrier's legs and arms.

Directions: Circle *Yes* if you agree with the statement and *No* if you disagree.

Yes No 1. The owner, animal control officer, or a police officer should kill the dog, decapitate its head, and send the head to a health department laboratory for a rabies analysis.

Yes No 2. In most parts of the United States, a dog usually does not have to be killed, but does need to be confined and observed for 10 days for rabies.

Yes No 3. The victim should receive medical care any time the skin is broken by an animal bite.

Yes No 4. Bleeding can usually be controlled using direct pressure.

Yes No 5. A first aider should close the wound with tape.

Answers: 1. No; 2. Yes; 3. Yes; 4. Yes; 5. No

▶ Check Your Knowledge

Directions: Circle *Yes* if you agree with the statement and *No* if you disagree.

Yes No 1. Report animal bites to the police or animal control officers.

Yes No 2. Apply cold or ice over a snakebite.

Yes No 3. Use the "cut-and-suck" method for a snakebite.

Yes No 4. Snakes have been known to bite more than once.

Yes No 5. Apply a cold or ice pack over an insect sting or a suspected spider bite.

Yes No 6. A baking soda paste can help reduce the itching and swelling from an insect sting.

Yes No 7. A victim's doctor-prescribed epinephrine injector may have to be used if the victim has a life-threatening reaction to an insect sting.

Yes No 8. Spider bite antivenin is available only for black widow spider bites, and not all victims need it.

Yes No 9. Victims allergic to insect stings should have epinephrine, which can be injected in cases of severe allergic reactions.

Yes No 10. Applying a blown-out, glowing match head or heated needle will cause an embedded tick to back out of a victim's skin.

Answers: 1. Yes; 2. No; 3. No; 4. Yes; 5. Yes; 6. Yes; 7. Yes; 8. Yes; 9. Yes; 10. No

Cold-Related Emergencies

▶ Environments

When exposed to very cold environments, the body may become overwhelmed. Cold exposure may cause injury to parts of the body by freezing (eg, frostbite) or to the body as a whole (eg, hypothermia).

Frostbite occurs only when the air temperature is below freezing (32° F) **Figure 15-1A, B**. Freezing limited to the skin surface is called *frostnip*. Freezing that extends deeper through the skin and into the flesh is called *frostbite*. Although hypothermia can occur in subfreezing temperatures, it can also happen in above-freezing temperatures—indoors or even on a summer day.

▶ Recognizing Frostnip

Frostnip is caused by water freezing on the surface of the skin. The skin becomes reddened and possibly swollen. Although frostnip is painful, there usually is no further damage after rewarming. Repeated frostnip in the same spot can dry the skin, causing it to crack and to become sensitive. It is difficult to tell the difference between frostnip and frostbite. Frostnip should be taken seriously because it may be the first sign of impending frostbite.

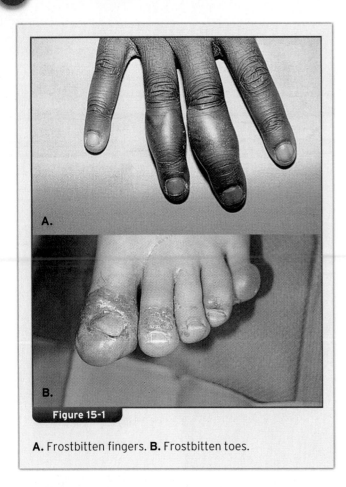

A. Frostbitten fingers. **B.** Frostbitten toes.

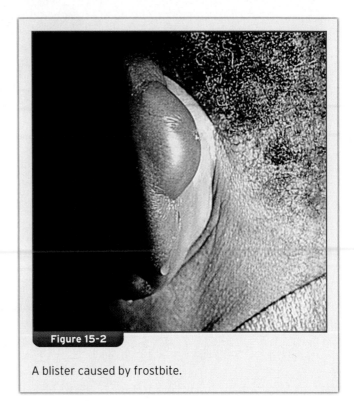

Figure 15-2

A blister caused by frostbite.

Care for Frostnip

To treat frostnip:

1. Gently warm the affected area by placing it against a warm body part (eg, put bare hands under the armpits or on the stomach or blow warm air on the area).
2. Do not rub the area. After rewarming, the affected area may be red and tingling.

▶ Recognizing Frostbite

Frostbite occurs when temperatures drop below freezing. Frostbite mainly affects the feet, hands, ears, and nose. These areas do not contain large heat-producing muscles and are some distance from the body's heat-generating sources. The most severe consequences of frostbite are gangrene and amputation.

The severity and extent of frostbite are difficult to judge until hours after thawing, although before thawing it can be classified as *superficial* or *deep*. Even physicians have to wait until thawing has occurred before they can judge the extent of the injury.

The signs and symptoms of superficial frostbite are:
- Skin color is white, waxy, or grayish-yellow.

- The affected part feels very cold and numb. There may be tingling, stinging, or aching sensations.
- The skin surface feels stiff or crusty, and the underlying tissue feels soft when depressed gently and firmly.

Deep frostbite is indicated by the following signs and symptoms:
- The affected part feels cold, hard, and solid and cannot be depressed.
- The affected part is cold, with pale, waxy skin.
- A painfully cold part suddenly stops hurting.
- Blisters may appear after rewarming **Figure 15-2**.

After a part has thawed, frostbite can be categorized by degrees, similar to the burn classifications (eg, first-, second-, or third-degree burn).

Care for Frostbite

Frostbite injuries require the following first aid treatment:

1. Get the victim out of the cold and into a warm place.
2. Remove any clothing or constricting items that could impair blood circulation (eg, rings).
3. Seek immediate medical care.
4. Place dry, sterile gauze between toes and the fingers to absorb moisture and to keep them from sticking together **Figure 15-3**.
5. Slightly elevate the affected part to reduce pain and swelling.

Frostbite

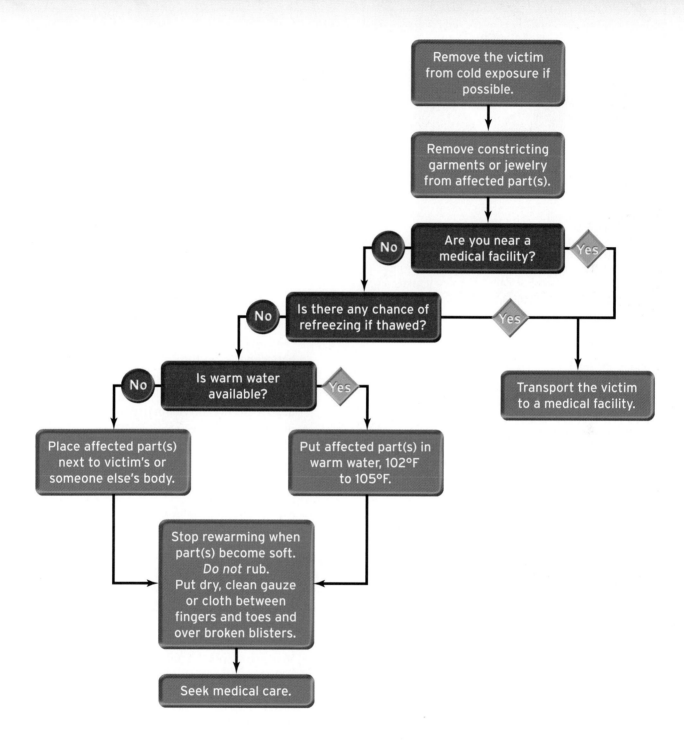

Remove the victim from cold exposure if possible.

↓

Remove constricting garments or jewelry from affected part(s).

↓

Are you near a medical facility?

No → / Yes →

No ↓

Is there any chance of refreezing if thawed?

Yes →

Transport the victim to a medical facility.

No ↓

Is warm water available?

No → / Yes →

Place affected part(s) next to victim's or someone else's body.

Put affected part(s) in warm water, 102°F to 105°F.

Stop rewarming when part(s) become soft. *Do not* rub. Put dry, clean gauze or cloth between fingers and toes and over broken blisters.

↓

Seek medical care.

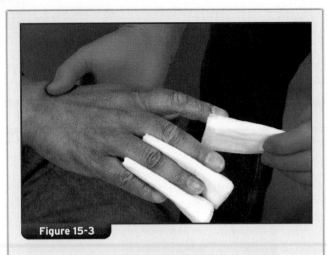

Figure 15-3

Place dry dressings between frostbitten fingers.

CAUTION

DO NOT rub or massage the frostbitten area.

DO NOT use the dry rewarming technique for frostbite (eg, victim's hands in your armpits), because it takes longer than the wet, rapid rewarming method to thaw frozen tissue.

FYI

Caring for Frostbite in a Remote Location

If the victim is in a remote or wilderness situation (more than 1 hour from medical care) and you have warm water, use the following wet, rapid rewarming method.

1. Place the frostbitten part in warm (102° F to 105° F) water. If you do not have a thermometer, pour some of the water over the inside of your arm or put your elbow into it to test that it is warm, not hot. Maintain water temperature by adding warm water as needed. Rewarming usually takes 20 to 40 minutes or until the tissues are soft. For ear or facial injuries, apply warm moist cloths, changing them frequently.

2. After thawing:
   - Treat victim as a "stretcher" case—the feet will be impossible to use after they are rewarmed.
   - Protect the affected area from contact with clothing and bedding.
   - Place dry, sterile gauze between the toes and the fingers to absorb moisture and to keep them from sticking together.
   - Slightly elevate the affected part to reduce pain and swelling.
   - Apply aloe vera gel to promote skin healing.
   - Give the victim ibuprofen to limit pain and inflammation.

▶ Recognizing Hypothermia

Body temperature falls when the body cannot produce heat as fast as it is being lost. <u>Hypothermia</u> is a life-threatening condition in which the body's core temperature falls below 95° F. Hypothermia can develop quickly (eg, cold water immersion) or gradually (eg, during prolonged exposure to a cold environment). The temperature does not have to be below freezing for hypothermia to occur.

The signs of hypothermia include the following:

- *Change in mental status.* This is one of the first symptoms of developing hypothermia. Examples are disorientation, apathy, and changes in personality, such as unusual aggressiveness.
- *Shivering.* Shivering is the body's first and most important defense against a falling body temperature. Shivering starts when the body temperature drops 1° F; it can produce more heat than many rewarming methods. As the core temperature continues to fall, however, shivering stops at about 90° F. Shivering also stops as body temperature rises. If shivering stops as responsiveness decreases, assume that the core temperature is falling.
- *Cool abdomen.* Place the back of your warm hand between the clothing and the victim's abdomen to assess the victim's temperature. When the victim's abdominal skin under clothing is cooler than your hand, consider the victim hypothermic until proven otherwise.
- *Low core body temperature.* The best indicator of hypothermia is a thermometer reading of the core body temperature, but normal thermometers do not register below 94° F, and therefore do not indicate whether the hypothermia is mild or severe. Rectal temperatures are seldom measured.

Recognizing Mild Hypothermia

Signs of mild hypothermia include the following:

- Vigorous, uncontrollable shivering.
- Victim has the "umbles"—grumbles, mumbles, fumbles, stumbles.
- Victim has cool or cold skin on the abdomen, chest, or back.
- Victim has a core body temperature above 90° F.

Care for Mild Hypothermia

Do the following to care for victims of mild hypothermia:

1. Stop further heat loss:
   - Get the victim out of the cold.
   - Handle the victim gently.

FYI

How Cold Is It?

In addition to cold, two other factors account for body heat loss: moisture and wind. Moisture—whether from rain, snow, or perspiration—speeds the conduction of heat away from the body.

Wind causes sizable amounts of body heat loss. If the thermometer reads 20° F and the wind speed is 20 mph, the exposure is comparable to 4° F. This is called the windchill factor. Use the following rough measures of wind speed: if you feel the wind on your face, wind speed is at least 10 mph; if small branches move or if dust or snow is raised, it is 20 mph; if large branches are moving, it is 30 mph; and if a whole tree bends, it is about 40 mph.

To determine the windchill factor:

1. Estimate the wind speed by checking for the aforementioned signs.
2. Look at an outdoor thermometer reading (in degrees Fahrenheit).
3. Match the estimated wind speed with the actual thermometer reading in the following table.

Source: National Weather Service.

Wind Chill Chart

Effective 11/01/01

Calm	40	35	30	25	20	15	10	5	0	-5	-10	-15	-20	-25	-30	-35	-40	-45
5	36	31	25	19	13	7	1	-5	-11	-16	-22	-28	-34	-40	-46	-52	-57	-63
10	34	27	21	15	9	3	-4	-10	-16	-22	-28	-35	-41	-47	-53	-59	-66	-72
15	32	25	19	13	6	0	-7	-13	-19	-26	-32	-39	-45	-51	-58	-64	-71	-77
20	30	24	17	11	4	-2	-9	-15	-22	-29	-35	-42	-48	-55	-61	-68	-74	-81
25	29	23	16	9	3	-4	-11	-17	-24	-31	-37	-44	-51	-58	-64	-71	-78	-84
30	28	22	15	8	1	-5	-12	-19	-26	-33	-39	-46	-53	-60	-67	-73	-80	-87
35	28	21	14	7	0	-7	-14	-21	-27	-34	-41	-48	-55	-62	-69	-76	-82	-89
40	27	20	13	6	-1	-8	-15	-22	-29	-36	-43	-50	-57	-64	-71	-78	-84	-91
45	26	19	12	5	-2	-9	-16	-23	-30	-37	-44	-51	-58	-65	-72	-79	-86	-93
50	26	19	12	4	-3	-10	-17	-24	-31	-38	-45	-52	-60	-67	-74	-81	-88	-95
55	25	18	11	4	-3	-11	-18	-25	-32	-39	-46	-54	-61	-68	-75	-82	-89	-97
60	25	17	10	3	-4	-11	-19	-26	-33	-40	-48	-55	-62	-69	-76	-84	-91	-98

Wind (mph)

Frostbite Times: ▨ 30 minutes ▨ 10 minutes ▨ 5 minutes

Wind Chill (°F) = $35.74 + 0.6215T - 35.75(V^{0.16}) + 0.4275T(V^{0.16})$

Where, T=Air Temperature (°F) V=Wind Speed (mph)

- Prevent heat loss by replacing wet clothing with dry clothing and placing insulation (eg, blankets, towels, pillows) beneath and over the victim. Cover the victim's head (50 to 80% of the body's heat loss is through the head).
- Keep the victim in a horizontal (flat) position. Do not raise the legs.
- Do not let the victim walk or exercise. Do not massage the victim's body.

2. Call 9-1-1 for immediate medical care. Remember that hypothermia is more common in urban settings than in victims found in the wilderness.

3. Do not attempt to stop shivering. Shivering generates large amounts of heat and will rewarm most victims. Heat packs etc. are not effective for rewarming a hypothermia victim.

CAUTION

If the victim is shivering, DO NOT stop it by adding heat (eg, with hot water bottles or heat packs). Shivering generates heat and will rewarm victims with mild hypothermia. Adding heat to the body should only be done at a hospital or when medical care is distant.

Recognizing Severe Hypothermia

The following signs indicate severe hypothermia:

- No shivering.
- Skin feels ice cold.
- Muscles can be stiff and rigid, similar to rigor mortis.

- Altered mental status—victim is not alert.
- Breathing slowly.
- Victim may appear to be dead.
- Victim has a core body temperature below 90° F.

Care for Severe Hypothermia

Care for someone with severe hypothermia by doing the following:

1. Stop further heat loss:
   - Get the victim out of the cold.
   - Handle the victim gently.
   - Prevent heat loss by replacing wet clothing with dry clothing and placing insulation (eg, blankets, towels, pillows,) beneath and over the victim. Cover the victim's head (50 to 80% of the body's heat loss is through the head).
   - Keep the victim in a horizontal (flat) position. Do not raise the legs.
   - Do not let the victim walk or exercise. Do not massage the victim's body.
2. Call 9-1-1 for immediate medical care.
3. When the victim is in a remote location and far from medical care, warm the victim by any available external heat (eg, body-to-body contact).

Hypothermia

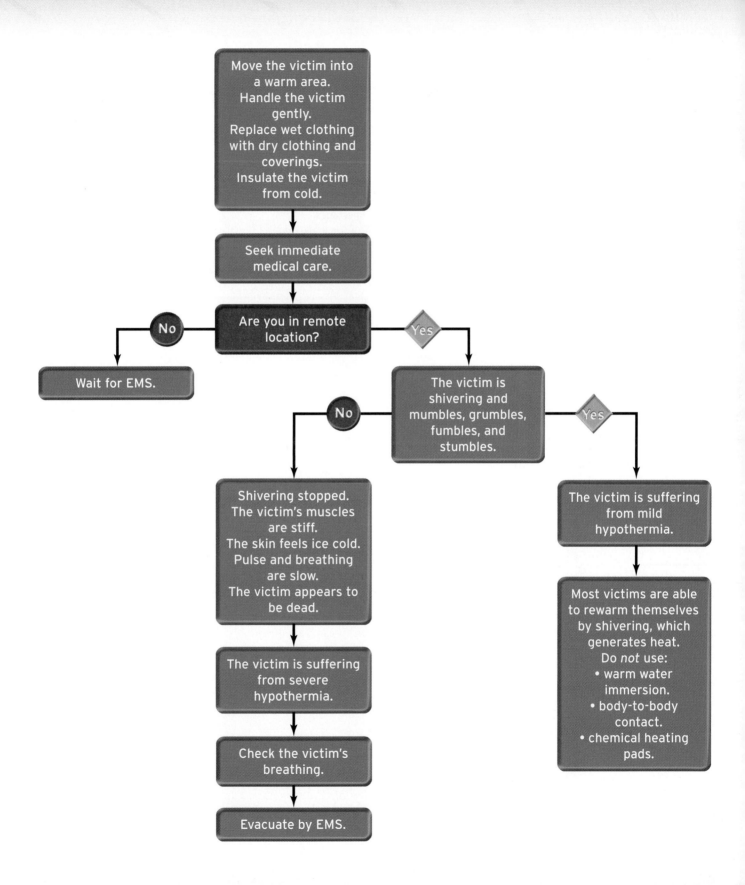

▶ Cold-Related Emergencies

What to Look For	What to Do

Frostbite

- White, waxy-looking skin
- Skin feels cold and numb (pain at first, followed by numbness)
- Blisters, which may appear after rewarming

1. Move victim to warm place.
2. Remove tight clothing or jewelry from injured part(s).
3. Place dry dressings between toes and/or fingers.
4. Seek medical care.

Hypothermia

- Mild
  - Uncontrollable shivering
  - Confusion, sluggishness
  - Cold skin even under clothing
- Severe
  - No shivering
  - Muscles stiff and rigid
  - Skin ice cold
  - Appears to be dead

1. Move victim to warm place.
2. Prevent heat loss by
   - Replacing wet clothing with dry clothing
   - Covering victim's head

Mild
1. Give warm, sugary beverages.
2. Do not add anything warm to the skin—let the shivering rewarm the body.

Severe
1. Do not rewarm unless in a very remote location.
2. Call 9-1-1.

▶ Ready for Review

- Frostbite occurs only when temperatures are below freezing.
- Frostbite requires medical care.
- Hypothermia can occur in subfreezing temperatures as well as above-freezing temperatures.
- Mild hypothermia is the most common and is identified by cold abdominal skin, shivering, and the "umbles"—the victim stumbles, fumbles, grumbles, and mumbles.
- Victims suffering severe hypothermia may appear to be dead.
- Shivering is the body's method to rewarm, and is the most effective way of rewarming in mild to moderate hypothermia.
- In severe hypothermia, seek immediate medical care, but if far from medical care apply external heat to victim.

▶ Vital Vocabulary

<u>frostbite</u> Tissue damage caused by extreme cold.

<u>frostnip</u> Irritation caused by water freezing on the skin surface.

<u>hypothermia</u> Life-threatening condition when the body's core temperature falls below 95° F.

▶ Assessment in Action

In subfreezing temperatures during a snowstorm, you find a stalled truck on a little-used road. Inside the truck is an elderly man, who tells you that his truck is out of gasoline and that when he tried to refill the truck's gas tank he dropped the gas can and some of the gasoline spilled onto his hands. He has been stranded for over 3 hours. The man complains of numbness where the gasoline was spilled on his hands. He did not know about a cabin about a quarter of a mile away.

Directions: Circle *Yes* if you agree with the statement and *No* if you disagree.

Yes   No   1. You suspect that the man's hands have frostbite.

Yes   No   2. You should check the man for hypothermia.

Yes   No   3. It is easy for most people to initially determine the extent and severity of frostbite.

Yes   No   4. Get the victim to the nearby cabin where his hands can be rewarmed.

Yes   No   5. Rubbing the affected area will restore blood circulation to the area.

Answers: 1. Yes; 2. Yes; 3. No; 4. Yes; 5. No

▶ Check Your Knowledge

Directions: Circle *Yes* if you agree with the statement and *No* if you disagree.

Yes   No   1. Rub or massage to rewarm a frostbitten part.

Yes   No   2. In a remote location, rapidly rewarm a frostbitten part by using warm water.

Yes   No   3. Placing frostbitten hands in another person's armpits is the best rewarming method to thaw frostbite.

Yes   No   4. When near a hospital, it's best to let medical personnel thaw the frostbitten part.

Yes   No   5. Add insulation (blankets) around and under the hypothermic victim.

Yes   No   6. Replace wet clothing with dry clothing.

Yes   No   7. Shivering is sufficient to rewarm a mildly hypothermic victim.

Yes   No   8. For severe hypothermia in a remote location and a day from medical care, use a rescuer's body heat to rewarm a victim.

Yes   No   9. Severe hypothermic victims should usually be transported to a hospital for rewarming.

Yes   No   10. Hypothermia requires below-freezing temperatures to develop.

Answers: 1. No; 2. Yes; 3. No; 4. Yes; 5. Yes; 6. Yes; 7. Yes; 8. Yes; 9. Yes; 10. No

Heat-Related Emergencies

▶ Heat-Related Disorders

A range of disorders can be classified as heat illnesses, including heat cramps, heat exhaustion, and heatstroke. Some of these conditions are common, but only heatstroke is life-threatening. Untreated heatstroke victims always die.

▶ Heat Cramps

Heat cramps are painful muscular spasms that happen suddenly, usually immediately after exertion. They usually involve the muscles in the back of the leg (calf and hamstring muscles) or the abdominal muscles. Some experts claim they are caused by salt depletion. Victims may be drinking fluids that do not have adequate salt content. However, other experts disagree, claiming that the typical American diet is heavy with salt.

Recognizing Heat Cramps

Heat cramps have the following characteristics:
- Painful muscle spasms that happen suddenly
- Affect the muscles in the back of the leg or abdomen
- Occur during or after physical exertion

Care for Heat Cramps

To relieve heat cramps (it may take several hours), follow these steps:

1. Rest in a cool place.
2. Drink lightly salted cool water (dissolve one-quarter teaspoon of salt in a quart of water) or a commercial sports drink.
3. Stretch the cramped muscle.
4. Try pinching the upper lip just below the nose (this is an accupuncture method).

▶ Heat Exhaustion

Heat exhaustion is caused by water or salt depletion, or both. Some experts believe that a better term would be *severe dehydration*. Heat exhaustion affects workers and athletes who do not drink enough fluids while working or exercising in hot environments. If untreated, it could develop into the more serious heatstroke.

Recognizing Heat Exhaustion

Heat exhaustion differs from heatstroke by having (1) no altered mental status and (2) skin that is not hot, but clammy. Heat exhaustion causes the following symptoms:

- Sweating
- Thirst
- Fatigue
- Flulike symptoms (headache and nausea)
- Shortness of breath
- Fast heart rate

Care for Heat Exhaustion

To care for heat exhaustion:

1. Move the victim immediately out of the heat to a cool place.
2. Give cool liquids, adding electrolytes (lightly salted water or a commercial sports drink) if plain water does not improve the victim's condition in 20 minutes. Do not give salt tablets; they can irritate the stomach and cause nausea and vomiting.
3. Raise the victim's legs 6 to 12 inches (keep the legs straight).
4. Remove excess clothing.
5. Sponge with cool water and fan the victim.
6. If you don't see any improvement within 30 minutes, seek medical care.

▶ Heatstroke

Two types of heatstroke exist: classic and exertional Table 16-1 . Classic heatstroke, also known as the *slow*

FYI

Heatstroke vs. Heat Exhaustion

Telling the difference between heat exhaustion and heatstroke is critical—the first is more common, but the second can be deadly. There are several ways to tell the difference between heat exhaustion and heatstroke. First, if the victim's body feels extremely hot when touched, suspect heatstroke. Another major mark of heatstroke is altered mental status (behavior), ranging from slight confusion and disorientation to coma. Between those extreme conditions, victims usually become irrational, agitated, or even aggressive, and may have seizures. In severe cases, the victim can go into a coma in less than an hour. The longer a coma lasts, the less the chance for survival. A third way to distinguish heatstroke from heat exhaustion is by rectal temperature. That is not very practical, however, because a responsive heatstroke victim may not cooperate. Taking a rectal temperature can be embarrassing to both the victim and the rescuer. Moreover, rectal thermometers are seldom available.

Table 16-1	Classic or Exertional Heatstroke?	
Characteristics	Classic	Exertional
Age group usually affected	Elderly	Males 15-45 years
Claims many victims at the same time	During heat waves	During athletic competition
Health status of victims	Chronically ill	Healthy and physically fit
Activity at the time of incident	Sedentary	Strenuous exercise
Medication use	Common	Usually none
Sweating	Absent	Often present (50% of victims)

cooker, may take days to develop. It is often seen during summer heat waves and typically affects the poor, the elderly, the chronically ill, alcoholics, or the obese. Because the elderly, who often have medical problems, are frequently afflicted, this type of heatstroke has a 50% death rate, even with medical care. It results from a combination of a hot environment and dehydration Table 16-2 . Exertional heatstroke is also more common in the summer. It is frequently seen in athletes, laborers, and military personnel, all of whom often sweat

Table 16-2   Heat Index

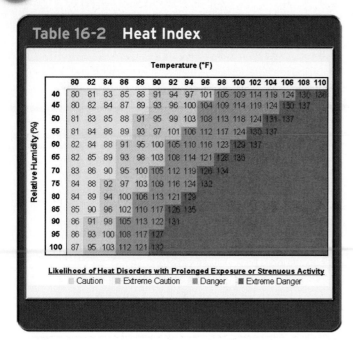

Temperature (°F)

Relative Humidity (%)	80	82	84	86	88	90	92	94	96	98	100	102	104	106	108	110
40	80	81	83	85	88	91	94	97	101	105	109	114	119	124	130	136
45	80	82	84	87	89	93	96	100	104	109	114	119	124	130	137	
50	81	83	85	88	91	95	99	103	108	113	118	124	131	137		
55	81	84	86	89	93	97	101	106	112	117	124	130	137			
60	82	84	88	91	95	100	105	110	116	123	129	137				
65	82	85	89	93	98	103	108	114	121	128	136					
70	83	86	90	95	100	105	112	119	126	134						
75	84	88	92	97	103	109	116	124	132							
80	84	89	94	100	106	113	121	129								
85	85	90	96	102	110	117	126	135								
90	86	91	98	105	113	122	131									
95	86	93	100	108	117	127										
100	87	95	103	112	121	132										

Likelihood of Heat Disorders with Prolonged Exposure or Strenuous Activity
▢ Caution   ▨ Extreme Caution   ▩ Danger   ▪ Extreme Danger

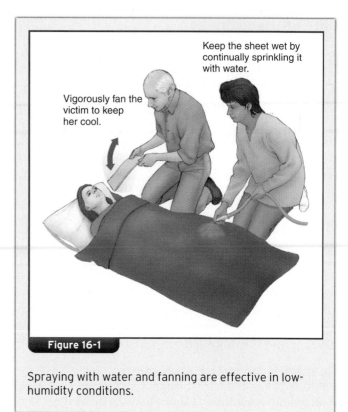

Vigorously fan the victim to keep her cool.

Keep the sheet wet by continually sprinkling it with water.

Figure 16-1

Spraying with water and fanning are effective in low-humidity conditions.

profusely. This type of heatstroke is known as the *fast cooker*. It affects healthy, active individuals who are working strenuously or playing in a warm environment. Because its rapid onset does not allow enough time for severe dehydration to occur, 50% of exertional heatstroke victims usually are sweating (classic heatstroke victims are not sweating.)

Recognizing Heatstroke

Signs of heatstroke include:
- Extremely hot skin when touched—usually dry, but can be wet in half of those with exertional heatstroke.
- Altered mental status ranging from slight confusion, agitation, and disorientation to unresponsiveness.

Care for Heatstroke

Heatstroke is a medical emergency and must be treated rapidly! Every minute delayed increases the likelihood of serious complications or death.

To care for heatstroke:
1. Seek immediate medical care by calling 9-1-1, even if the victim seems to be recovering.
2. Move the victim immediately to a cool place.
3. Remove all clothing down to the victim's underwear.
4. Keep the victim's head and shoulders slightly elevated.
5. The only way to prevent damage is to cool the victim quickly and by any means possible. Rapidly cool the victim by whatever means possible:
   - Spraying the victim with water and then fanning **Figure 16-1**. This method is not as effective in high-humidity (more than 75%) conditions.
   - Apply cool wet sheets or towels.
   - Place ice bags against the large veins in the groin, arm-pits, and sides of the neck to cool the body regardless of the humidity.

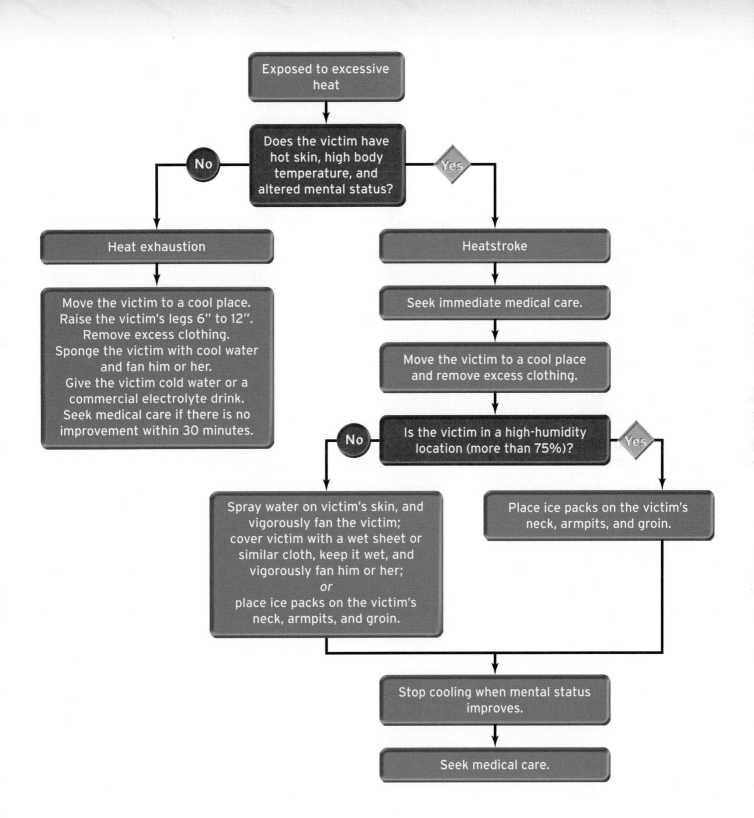

prep kit

▶ Ready for Review

- Given the right conditions, anyone can develop a heat illness.
- Heat illnesses range from heat cramps to heatstroke. Only heatstroke is life-threatening.
- Treat heat cramps by stretching the affected muscle and giving water or a commercial sports drink.
- Treat heat exhaustion, which may be better called *severe dehydration*, by applying cold towels to the body and giving water or a commercial sports drink.
- Two types of heatstroke exist: classic and exertional.
- Treat heatstroke as an emergency. Call 9-1-1 immediately for medical care. Cool the victim with whatever you have (eg, sprinkling and fanning the victim, placing ice packs against the armpits, side of neck, and groin).

▶ Vital Vocabulary

<u>heat cramps</u> Painful muscle spasms, often in the legs.

<u>heat exhaustion</u> Condition caused by the loss of the body's water and salt through excessive sweating.

<u>heatstroke</u> The body's heat-regulating ability becomes overwhelmed and ceases to function properly, resulting in an inability to sweat and a dangerously high body temperature.

▶ Assessment in Action

A teenager's summer job is mowing lawns for various companies in an industrial park. He is sweating heavily on a very hot, humid day. He complains about being very thirsty, nauseous, and having a headache.

Directions: Circle *Yes* if you agree with the statement and *No* if you disagree.

Yes	No	1. You suspect that he is suffering from a heat cramp.
Yes	No	2. Do not move him into a cooler place, because it will be a shock to the body.
Yes	No	3. Elevate his head 6 to 12 inches.
Yes	No	4. The victim probably does not need medical care unless there is no improvement in 30 minutes.
Yes	No	5. Give him a cool drink, such as a commercial sports drink or water.

Answers: **1.** No; **2.** No; **3.** No; **4.** Yes; **5.** Yes

▶ Check Your Knowledge

Directions: Circle *Yes* if you agree with the statement and *No* if you disagree.

Yes	No	1. For heat cramps, stretch a cramped muscle.
Yes	No	2. Salt tablets can be given to victims of any heat illness.
Yes	No	3. Move heat illness victims out of the heat to a cool place.
Yes	No	4. Heat exhaustion victims need immediate medical care—it's a life-threatening condition.
Yes	No	5. Heatstroke victims need immediate cooling by any means possible.
Yes	No	6. Apply rubbing alcohol on a heatstroke victim's skin for cooling.
Yes	No	7. If in high-humidity conditions, spray and fan the heatstroke victim.
Yes	No	8. Regardless of humidity, cold or ice packs applied to the neck, armpits, and groin helps to cool a heatstroke victim.
Yes	No	9. Exertional heatstroke is found in athletes, laborers, and military personnel.
Yes	No	10. Heat exhaustion can be described as severe dehydration.

Answers: **1.** Yes; **2.** No; **3.** Yes; **4.** No; **5.** Yes; **6.** No; **7.** No; **8.** Yes; **9.** Yes; **10.** Yes

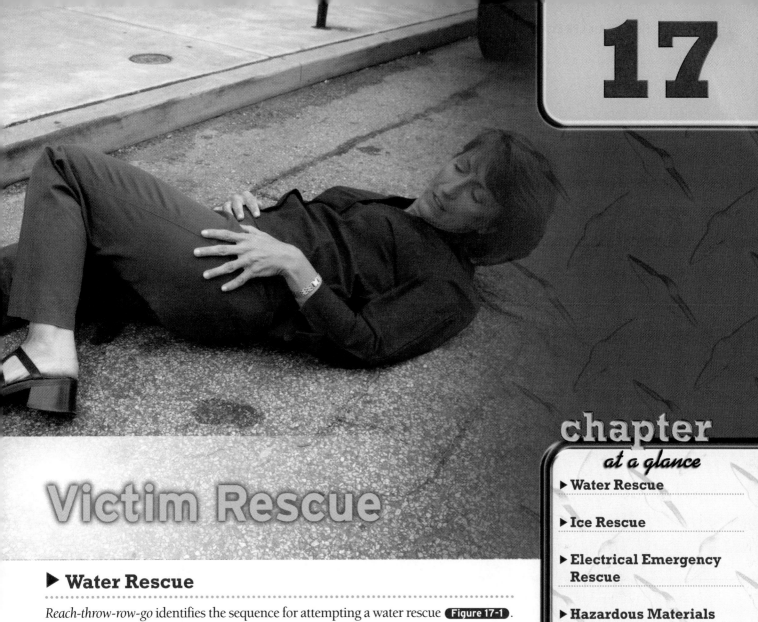

Victim Rescue

▶ Water Rescue

Reach-throw-row-go identifies the sequence for attempting a water rescue **Figure 17-1** . The first and simplest rescue technique is to reach for the victim. Reaching requires a lightweight pole, a ladder, a long stick, or any object that can be extended to the victim. Once you have your "reacher," secure your footing and have a bystander grab your belt or pants for stability. Secure yourself before reaching for the victim.

You can throw anything that floats—an empty picnic jug, an empty fuel or paint can, a life jacket, a floating cushion, a piece of wood, an inflated spare wheel— whatever is available. If there is a rope handy, tie it to the object to be thrown so you can pull the victim in, or, if you miss, you can retrieve the object and throw it again. The average untrained rescuer has a throwing range of about 50 feet.

If the victim is out of throwing range and there is a rowboat, canoe, motor boat, or boogie board nearby, you can try to row to the victim. Maneuvering these craft requires skills learned through practice. Wear a personal flotation device (PFD) for your own safety. To avoid capsizing, never pull the victim in over the side of a boat; pull over the stern (rear end).

If the reach-throw-row techniques are impossible and you are a capable swimmer trained in water lifesaving procedures, you can go to the drowning victim by swimming. Entering even calm water makes a swimming rescue difficult and hazardous. If you are grabbed by a victim and cannot escape, a good self-rescue technique is to take a deep breath and then allow yourself to sink under the surface. Victims will feel themselves being pulled under and almost always let go. All too often a would-be rescuer becomes a victim as well.

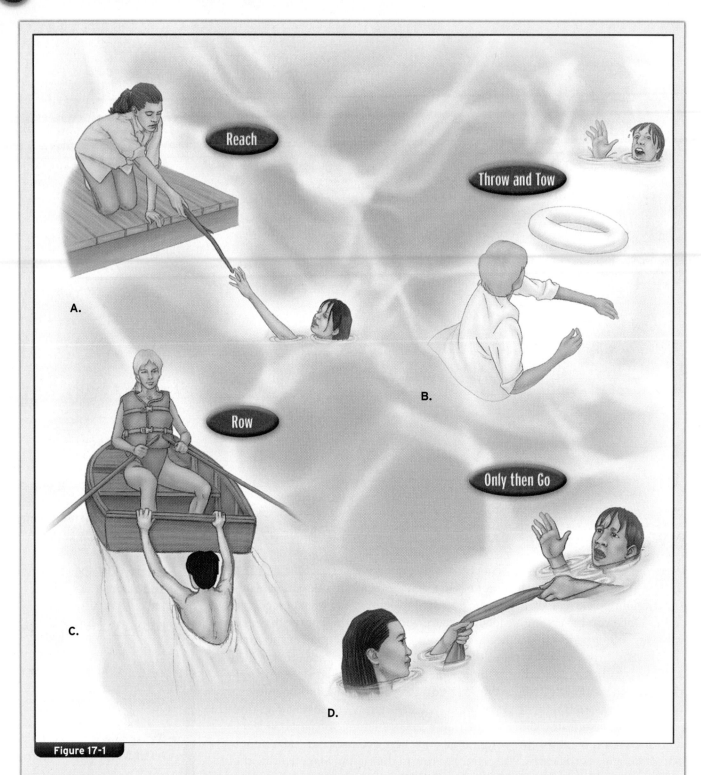

Figure 17-1

Basic rules of water rescue. **A.** Reach for the person from shore. If you cannot reach the person from shore, wade closer.
B. If an object that floats is available, throw it to the person. **C.** Use a boat if one is available. **D.** If you must swim to the
person, use a towel or board for him or her to hold onto. Do not let the person grab you.

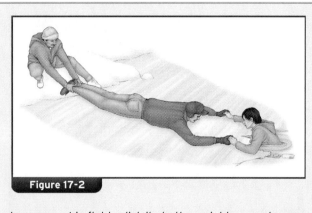

Figure 17-2

Ice rescue: Lie flat to distribute the weight over a larger surface area.

CAUTION

DO NOT swim to and grasp a drowning person unless you are trained to make the rescue.

▶ Ice Rescue

If a person has fallen through ice near the shore, extend a pole or throw a line with a floatable object attached to it. Once the person has hold of the object, pull him or her toward the shore or the edge of the ice.

If the person has fallen through the ice away from the shore and you cannot reach him or her with a pole or a throwing line, lie flat and push a ladder, plank, or similar object ahead of you **Figure 17-2**. You can tie a rope to a spare tire and the other end to an anchor point, lie flat, and push the wheel ahead of you. Pull the person ashore or to the edge of the ice.

CAUTION

DO NOT go near broken ice without support.

▶ Electrical Emergency Rescue

Electrical injuries can be devastating. Just a mild shock can cause serious internal injuries. A current of 1,000 volts or more is considered high voltage, but even the 110 volts of household current can be deadly.

When a person gets an electric shock, electricity enters the body at the point of contact and travels along the path of least resistance (nerves and blood vessels). The current travels rapidly, generating heat and causing destruction.

Most indoor electrocutions are caused by faulty electrical equipment or careless use of electrical appliances. Before you touch the victim, turn off the electricity at the circuit breaker, fuse box, or outside switch box or unplug the appliance (if the plug is undamaged). If the electrocution involves high-voltage power lines, the power must be turned off before anyone approaches a victim. If you approach a victim and feel a tingling sensation in your legs and lower body, stop. You are on energized ground, and an electrical current is entering one foot, passing through your lower body, and leaving through the other foot. If that happens, raise one foot off the ground, turn around, and hop to a safe place. Wait for trained personnel with the proper equipment to cut the wires or disconnect them. If a power line has fallen over a car, tell the driver and passengers to stay in the car. A victim should try to jump out of the car only if an explosion or fire threatens, and then without making contact with the car or the wire.

CAUTION

DO NOT touch an appliance or the victim until the current is off.

DO NOT try to move downed wires.

DO NOT use any object, even dry wood (eg, broomstick, tools, chair, stool) to separate the victim from the electrical source.

▶ Hazardous Materials Incidents

At almost any highway crash scene, there is the potential danger of hazardous chemicals. The following may indicate the presence of hazardous materials:

- Look for warning signs on the vehicle (eg, "explosive," "flammable," "corrosive"). If you are unable to read the placard or labels, do not move closer and risk exposure. If you are able to read the placard with the naked eye, you may be too close and should consider moving farther away. **Figure 17-3** shows hazardous materials warning placards, and **Figure 17-4** shows various warning labels.
- Watch for a leak or spill from a tank, container, truck, or railroad car with or without hazardous material placards or labels.
- A strong, noxious odor can denote a hazardous material.
- A cloud or strange-looking smoke from the escaping substance "says" stay away.

Stay well away and upwind from the area. Only those who are specially trained in handling hazardous materials and who have the proper equipment should be in the area.

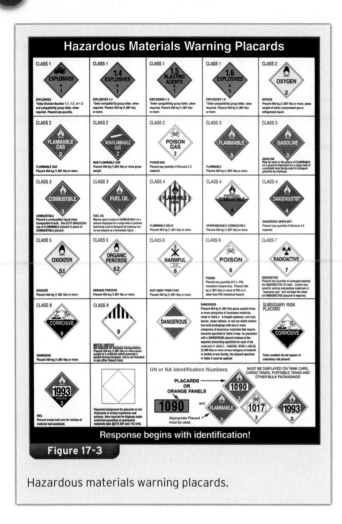

Figure 17-3

Hazardous materials warning placards.

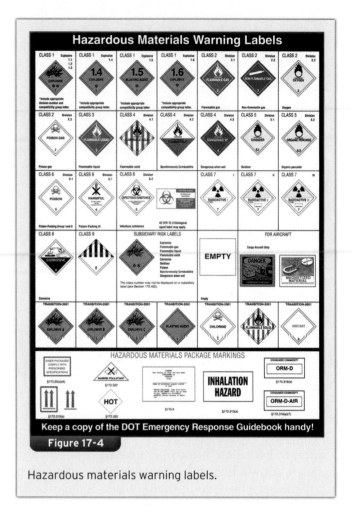

Figure 17-4

Hazardous materials warning labels.

▶ Motor Vehicle Crashes

You are legally obligated to stop and give help when you are involved in a motor vehicle crash. If you come to a crash shortly after it happens, the law does not require you to stop, although it might be argued that you have a moral responsibility to render any aid you can. If you encounter a motor vehicle crash, you should:

1. Stop and park your vehicle well off the highway or road and out of active traffic lanes. Park at least five car lengths from the crash. If the police have taken charge, do not stop unless you are asked to do so. If the police or other emergency vehicles have not arrived, call or send someone to call 9-1-1 or the local emergency number as soon as possible. Ways to call include:
   - Find a pay phone or roadside emergency phone.
   - Use a cellular phone.
   - Ask to use a phone at a nearby house or business.

2. Turn on your vehicle's emergency hazard flashers. Raise the hood of your vehicle to draw more attention to the scene.

3. Make sure everyone on the scene is safe.
   - Ask the driver(s) to turn off the ignition or turn it off yourself.
   - Ask bystanders to stand well off the roadway.
   - Place flares or reflectors 250 to 500 feet behind the crash scene to warn oncoming drivers of the crash. Do not ignite flares around leaking gasoline or diesel fuel.

4. If the driver or passenger is unresponsive or might have spinal injuries, use your hands to stabilize the head and neck.

5. Check and keep monitoring breathing. Treat any life-threatening injuries.

6. Whenever possible, wait for EMS personnel to extricate the victims from vehicles, because they have training and the proper equipment. In most cases, keep the victims stabilized inside the vehicle.

7. Allow the EMS ambulance to take victims to the hospital.

CAUTION

DO NOT rush to get victims out of a car that has been in a crash. Contrary to opinion, most vehicle crashes do not involve fire, and most vehicles stay in an upright position.

DO NOT move or allow victims to move unless there is an immediate danger, such as fire or oncoming traffic. Treat victims as though every bone in their bodies is broken.

DO NOT transport victims in your car or any other bystander's vehicle.

▶ Fires

If you encounter a fire, you should:

1. Get all the people out fast.
2. Call 9-1-1.

Then—and only then—if the fire is small, and if your own escape route is clear, should you fight the fire yourself with a fire extinguisher. You may be able to put out the fire or at least hold damage to a minimum.

To use a fire extinguisher, aim directly at whatever is burning and sweep across it. Extinguishers expel their contents quickly, in 8 to 25 seconds for most home models containing dry chemicals.

CAUTION

DO NOT get trapped while fighting a fire. Always stay close to an open door so you can exit if the fire gets too big.

▶ Confined Spaces

A confined space is an area not intended for human occupancy that also has the potential for containing or accumulating a dangerous atmosphere. There are three types of confined spaces: below ground, ground level, and above ground. Below-ground confined spaces include manholes, below-ground utility vaults, storage tanks, old mines, cisterns, and wells. Ground-level confined spaces include industrial tanks and farm storage silos. Above-ground confined spaces include water towers and storage tanks.

An accident in a confined space demands immediate action. If someone who enters a confined space signals for help or becomes unconscious, follow these steps to help:

1. Call 9-1-1 for immediate help.
2. Do not rush in to help.
3. When help arrives, try to rescue the victim without entering the space.

4. If rescue from the outside cannot be done, allow trained and properly equipped (respiratory protection plus safety harnesses or lifelines) rescuers to enter the space and remove the victim.
5. Once the victim is removed, provide care.

▶ Triage: What to Do with Multiple Victims

You may encounter emergency situations in which there are two or more victims. This often happens in multiple-car accidents or disasters. After making a quick scene survey, decide who must be cared for and transported first. This process of prioritizing or classifying injured victims is called triage. The word triage is derived from the French word trier, which means "to sort." The goal is to do the greatest good for the greatest number of victims.

A variety of systems are used to identify care and transportation priorities. To find those needing immediate care for life-threatening conditions, first tell all victims who can get up and walk to move to a specific area. Victims who can get up and walk rarely have life-threatening injuries. These victims ("walking wounded") are classified as "delayed priority" (see below). Do not force a victim to move if he or she complains of pain.

Find the life-threatened victims by performing the initial check on all remaining victims. Go to motionless victims first. You must move quickly (spend less than 60 seconds with each victim) from one victim to the next until all have been assessed. Classify victims according to the following care and transportation priorities:

1. *Immediate care.* Victim needs immediate care and transport to medical care as soon as possible:
   - Breathing difficulties
   - Severe bleeding
   - Severe burns
   - Signs of shock
   - Unresponsiveness
2. *Delayed care.* Care and transport can be delayed up to 1 hour:
   - Burns without airway problems
   - Major or multiple bone or joint injuries
   - Back injuries with or without suspected spinal cord damage
3. *Walking wounded.* Care and transportation can be delayed up to 3 hours:
   - Minor fractures
   - Minor wounds
4. *Dead.* Victim is obviously dead or unlikely to survive because of the type and extent of the injuries. This includes most cases of cardiac arrest due to injury.

Do not become involved in treating the victims at this point, but ask knowledgeable bystanders to care for immediate life-threatening problems (ie, bleeding control).

Reassess victims regularly for changes in their condition. Only after victims with immediate life-threatening conditions receive care should those with less-serious conditions be given care.

Later, you will usually be relieved when more highly trained emergency personnel arrive on the scene. You may then be asked to provide first aid, to help move victims, or to help with ambulance or helicopter transportation.

▶ Moving Victims

A victim should not be moved until he or she is ready for transportation to a hospital, if required. All necessary first aid should be provided first. A victim should be moved only if there is an immediate danger:

- There is a fire or danger of fire.
- Explosives or other hazardous materials are involved.
- It is impossible to protect the scene from hazards.
- It is impossible to gain access to other victims in the situation (eg, a vehicle) who need life-saving care.

A cardiac-arrest victim is usually moved unless he or she is already on the ground or floor, because CPR must be performed on a firm surface.

CAUTION

DO NOT move a victim unless you absolutely have to, such as when the victim is in immediate danger or must be moved to shelter while waiting for the EMS to arrive.

Emergency Moves

The major danger in moving a victim quickly is the possibility of aggravating a spinal injury. In an emergency, every effort should be made to pull the victim in the direction of the long axis of the body to provide as much protection to the spinal cord as possible. If victims are on the floor or ground, you can drag them away from the scene by using various techniques (Figure 17-5) through (Figure 17-18).

Nonemergency Moves

All injured parts should be stabilized before and during moving. If rapid transportation is not needed, it is helpful to find another person about the same size as the injured person to help move the victim.

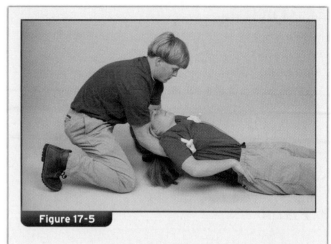

Figure 17-5

Shoulder drag. Use for short distances over a rough surface; stabilize the victim's head with your forearms.

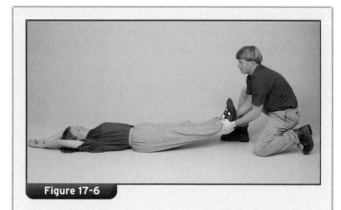

Figure 17-6

Ankle drag. This is the fastest method for a short distance on a smooth surface.

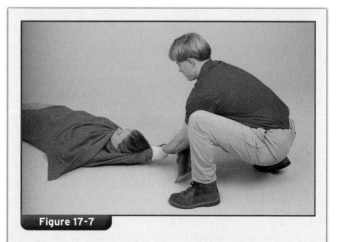

Figure 17-7

Blanket pull. Roll the victim onto a blanket, and pull from behind the victim's head.

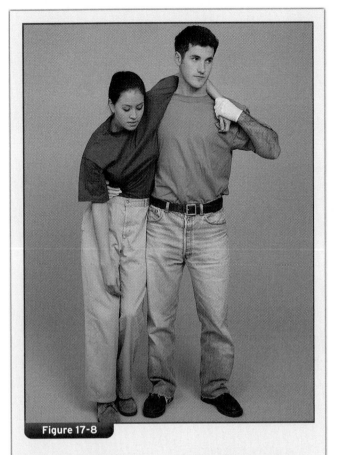

Figure 17-8

Human crutch (one person helps the victim to walk).
If one leg is injured, help the victim to walk on the good
leg while you support the injured side.

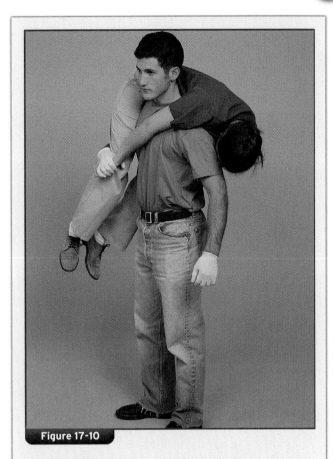

Figure 17-10

Fire fighter's carry. If the victim's injuries permit, you
can travel longer distances if you carry the victim over
your shoulder.

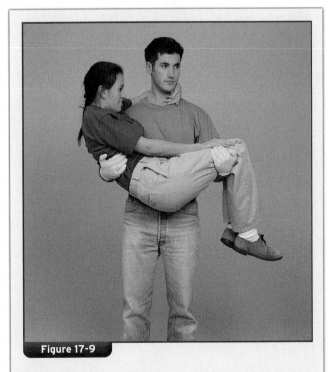

Figure 17-9

Cradle carry. Use this method for children and lightweight
adults who cannot walk.

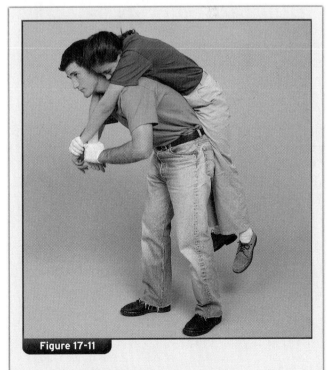

Figure 17-11

Pack-strap carry. When injuries make the fire fighter's
carry unsafe, this method is better for longer distances.

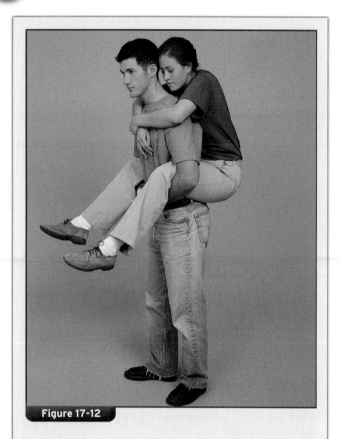

Figure 17-12

Piggyback carry. Use this method when the victim cannot walk but can use the arms to hang on to the rescuer.

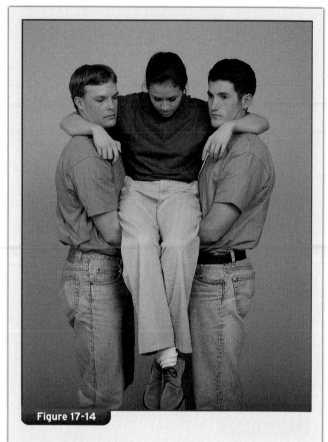

Figure 17-14

Two-handed seat carry.

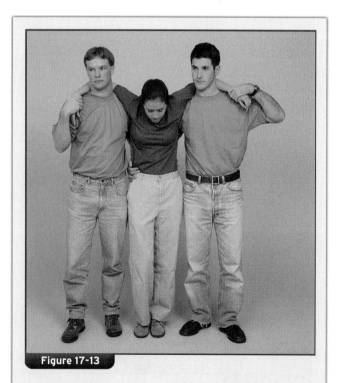

Figure 17-13

Two-person assist. This method is similar to the human crutch.

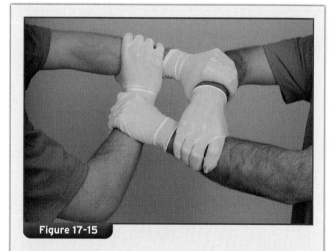

Figure 17-15

Four-handed seat carry. This is the easiest two-person carry when no equipment is available and the victim cannot walk but can use the arms to hang onto the rescuers.

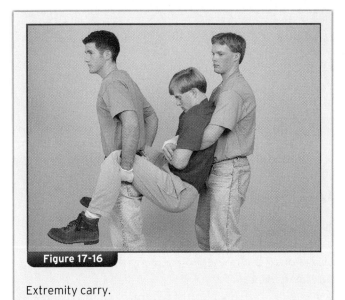

Figure 17-16

Extremity carry.

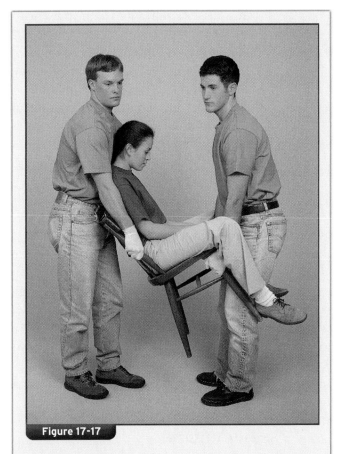

Figure 17-17

Chair carry. This method is useful for a narrow passage or up or down stairs. Use a sturdy chair that can take the victim's weight.

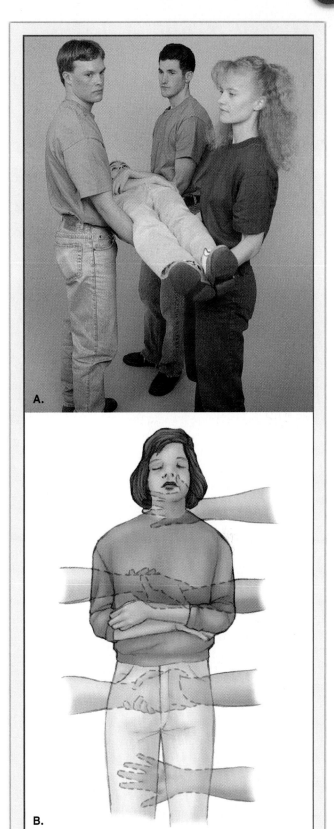

A.

B.

Figure 17-18

Hammock carry. **A.** Three to six people stand on alternate sides of the injured person; and **B.** link hands beneath the victim.

prep kit

▶ Ready for Review

- *Reach-throw-row-go* identifies the sequence for attempting a water rescue.
- If a person has fallen through the ice near the shore, extend a pole or throw a line with a floatable object attached to it.
- Almost any highway crash scene involves the potential danger of hazardous chemicals.
- When involved in a motor vehicle crash, most state laws require the driver to stop and render care.
- Should you encounter a fire, you should get all people out fast and call 9-1-1.
- A confined space is any area not intended for human occupancy that may have or develop a dangerous atmosphere.
- The goal of triage is to do the greatest good for the greatest number of victims.
- The major danger in moving a victim quickly is the possibility of aggravating a spinal injury.

▶ Vital Vocabulary

triage The sorting of patients into groups according to the severity of injuries. Used to determine priorities for treatment and transport.

▶ Assessment in Action

You see a single car leave the highway and crash into an electrical power line pole, knocking down some of the high-voltage power lines. One victim is ejected from the car, and another remains in the car yelling for help.
Directions: Circle *Yes* if you agree with the statement and *No* if you disagree.

Yes   No   1. You should go first to the victim in the car because he or she is pleading for help.

Yes   No   2. If one of the victims is in contact with the high-voltage power line, use a dry tree branch to move the electrical line.

Yes   No   3. Most state laws require a driver of another car who witnessed a crash, even though he or she was not involved in the crash, to stop and render care.

Yes   No   4. Always suspect a spinal injury in motor vehicle crashes.

Yes   No   5. Turning on your vehicle's emergency hazard flashers and raising the hood of your vehicle when you stop to help at a crash scene draws attention to the scene.

Answers: 1. No; 2. No; 3. No; 4. Yes; 5. Yes

▶ Check Your Knowledge

Directions: Circle *Yes* if you agree with the statement and *No* if you disagree.

Yes   No   1. You should attempt to move downed power lines away from a victim, using a broom or other wooden object.

Yes   No   2. Strong, unusual odors or clouds of vapor are possible indications of the presence of hazardous materials.

Yes   No   3. To keep from getting trapped while attempting to extinguish a fire, you should always keep a door behind you for rapid exit.

Yes   No   4. When triaging victims, breathing difficulties are classified as urgent-care priorities.

Yes   No   5. A major concern in moving a victim quickly is the possibility of aggravating a spinal injury.

Yes   No   6. *Reach-throw-row-go* represents the safe order for executing a water rescue.

Yes   No   7. In most states, you are not legally obligated to stop and give help when you are involved in a motor vehicle crash.

Yes   No   8. You can throw anything that floats (eg, empty picnic jug, wood) to a distressed in-the-water person.

Yes   No   9. A PFD represents a life jacket also known as a *personal flotation device*.

Yes   No   10. Before helping a victim being electrocuted in a home, turn off the electricity.

Answers: 1. No; 2. Yes; 3. Yes; 4. Yes; 5. Yes; 6. No; 7. Yes; 8. Yes; 9. Yes; 10. Yes

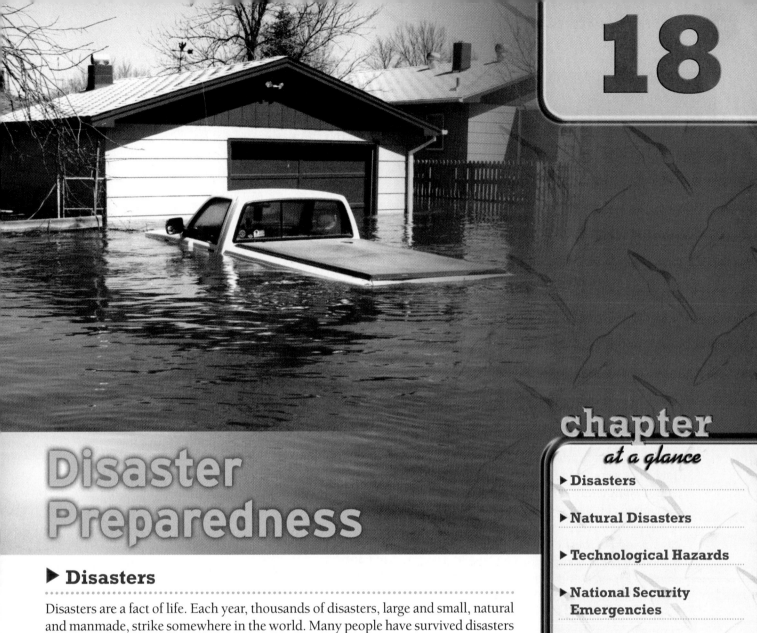

Disaster Preparedness

▶ Disasters

Disasters are a fact of life. Each year, thousands of disasters, large and small, natural and manmade, strike somewhere in the world. Many people have survived disasters thanks to good luck and willpower. But that is not enough. Training about disasters needs to be modified from a "nice-to-know" to a "must-know" requirement.

This chapter presents valuable information about disasters. The information is adapted from US government documents provided by the Federal Emergency Management Agency (FEMA), The Department of Homeland Security, the National Weather Service, and the US Geological Survey.

▶ Natural Disasters

Natural disasters such as earthquakes, floods, hurricanes, and tornados claim many lives each year. Becoming informed about the dangers of natural disasters and the steps you can take to protect yourself and others can help to minimize the death toll.

Earthquakes

An earthquake is a sudden, rapid shaking of the earth caused by the breaking and shifting of rock deep beneath the earth's surface. This shaking can cause buildings and bridges to collapse; disrupt gas, electric, and phone service; and sometimes trigger landslides, avalanches, flash floods, fires, and huge, destructive ocean waves (tsunamis). Earthquakes can occur at any time of the year **Figure 18-1**.

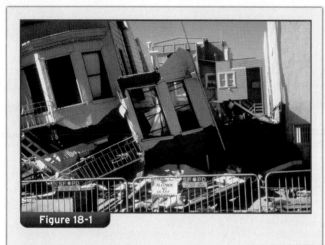

Figure 18-1

Devastation resulting from the California earthquake that crippled San Francisco in 1989.

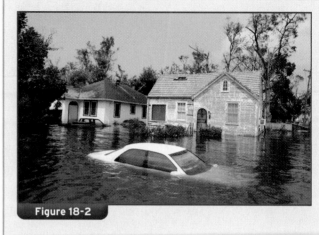

Figure 18-2

Hurricane Katrina caused massive floods in New Orleans.

Safety During an Earthquake

Follow these safety guidelines if you experience an earthquake:

- If you are indoors, take cover under a sturdy desk, table, bench, or against an inside wall. If the earthquake is severe, crouch next to a large, sturdy object, such as a refrigerator or file cabinet. Should the ceiling collapse, a triangle of space next to the object will provide a safe place. Stay away from glass, windows, outside doors, walls, and anything that could fall. If there is not a table or desk nearby, cover your face and head with your arms and crouch down. Stay inside until the shaking has stopped and you are sure exiting is safe. It is dangerous to try to leave a building during an earthquake, because objects can fall on you. Beware of aftershocks and follow the same precautions.
- If you are in bed, stay there and protect your head with a pillow, unless you are under a heavy light or fan fixture that could fall. If the earthquake is severe, get on the floor next to, but not under, the bed. This will also provide a safe space if the ceiling collapses.
- If you are in a high-rise building, expect the fire alarms and sprinklers to go off during an earthquake. Do not use the elevators; use the stairs.
- If you are outdoors, find a clear spot away from buildings, trees, streetlights, and power lines. Drop to the ground and stay there until the shaking stops.
- If you are in a vehicle, pull over and stay there with your seatbelt fastened until the shaking has stopped. If the earthquake is severe and you are underneath a highway overpass, exit your car and lie next to, but not underneath your vehicle. The

falling debris may crush the roof of the car, but beside the car will be a safe place for you to stay until help arrives.
- If you are trapped in debris do not panic. Move carefully.
  - Do not light a match.
  - Do not move about or kick up dust.
  - Cover your mouth with a handkerchief or clothing.
  - Tap on a pipe or wall so rescuers can locate you.

Floods

With the exception of fire, floods are the most common and widespread of all natural disasters. Most communities have experienced some type of flooding after heavy spring rains, heavy thunderstorms, or winter snow thaws **Figure 18-2** .

Pay attention to flash flood warnings even if skies are clear in your location, because run-off can occur from storms miles away. Be especially aware of storms in hills above you. Flash floods occur when heavy rain causes run-off into channels and low-lying areas. The flood can be very fast and occur miles from the rain, often catching people off guard.

Safety During a Flood

Follow these safety guidelines if conditions exist that could cause a flood:

- Be aware of the likelihood of flooding in your area. If there is any possibility of a flood or flash flood, move immediately to higher ground. Be aware of streams, drainage channels, canyons, and other areas known to flood suddenly.
- Listen to radio or television stations for local information.

- If local authorities issue a flood watch, prepare to evacuate:
  - Secure your home, if you have time. Move essential items to upper floors.
  - If instructed, turn off utilities at the main switches or valves. Disconnect electrical appliances. Do not touch electrical equipment if you are wet or standing in water.
  - If you are not evacuating, you still need to prepare for the worst. If you do not have access to adequate bottled water, you can fill the bathtub with water in case water becomes contaminated or services are cut off. Before filling the tub, sterilize it with a diluted bleach solution (1 part bleach: 10 parts water).
- Do not walk through moving water. Six inches of moving water can knock you off your feet. Use a stick or pole to check the firmness of the ground and water depth in front of you.
- Do not drive into flooded areas. A foot of water can float a vehicle. Two feet of water can carry away most vehicles, including sport utility vehicles (SUVs) and pickups.
- If flood water rises around your car, abandon the car and move to higher ground, but only if you can do so safely.

Heat Waves (Extreme Heat)

In extreme heat and high humidity, cooling of the body by evaporation is slowed and the body must work extra hard to maintain normal temperature **Figure 18-3**. People living in urban areas may be at greater risk from the effects of a prolonged heat wave than those living in rural areas. Asphalt and concrete store heat longer and gradually release heat at night.

Safety During a Heat Wave

Follow these safety guidelines if you experience a heat wave emergency:

- Stay in the coolest available location. Stay indoors as much as possible. If air conditioning is not available, stay on the lowest floor, out of the sunshine. Circulate air with a fan and use cool wet cloths to help keep your body temperature down.
- Drink plenty of water regularly, even if you do not feel thirsty.
- Avoid alcoholic beverages, because they cause further dehydration.
- Never leave children or pets alone in vehicles.
- Dress in loose-fitting clothes. Lightweight, light-colored clothing reflects heat and sunlight and helps maintain normal body temperature.

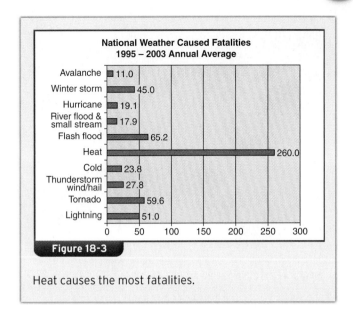

Figure 18-3

Heat causes the most fatalities.

- Protect the face and head by wearing a wide-brimmed hat.
- Avoid too much sunshine. Sunburn slows the skin's ability to cool itself.
- Avoid strenuous work during the warmest part of the day.
- Spend at least 2 hours of the day in an air-conditioned place. If your home is not air conditioned, consider spending the warmest part of the day in public buildings (eg, libraries, movie theaters, shopping malls).
- Check on family, friends, and neighbors who do not have air conditioning and who spend much of their time alone. Refer to Chapter 16 for first aid procedures for heat-related emergencies (eg, heatstroke, heat exhaustion, heat cramps).

Hurricanes

A hurricane is a tropical storm with winds that have reached a constant speed of at least 74 miles per hour. As a hurricane nears land, it can bring torrential rains, high winds, and flooding from the ocean, called storm surges. All Atlantic and Gulf of Mexico coastal areas are subject to hurricanes or tropical storms. August and September are peak months of hurricane activity during the storm season, which lasts from June to November **Figure 18-4**.

Safety During a Hurricane

Follow these safety guidelines if you experience the threat of a hurricane:

- Listen to a radio or television newscasts. If a hurricane "watch" is issued, you usually have 24 to 36 hours before the hurricane hits land.
- Secure your home. Close any storm shutters. Secure outdoor objects or bring them indoors.

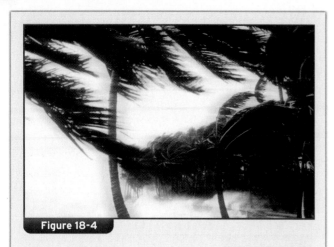

Figure 18-4

Hurricanes are among the most costly and dangerous disasters.

Attach boards to window frames or tape windows to prevent or reduce risk of broken glass. Park any cars remaining at home along the side of the house. Make sure that all vehicles have a full tank of gas.

- If you are not evacuating, you still need to prepare for the worst. Gather several days' supply of water and food for each household member. If you do not have access to adequate bottled water, fill the bathtub with water in case water becomes contaminated or services are cut off. Before filling the tub, sterilize it with a diluted bleach solution (1 part bleach: 10 parts water).
- If you are evacuating, prepare backpacks to take your disaster supplies with you to the shelter.
- When preparing to evacuate, fuel your vehicle and review evacuation routes. If instructed, turn off utilities at the main valves or switches before departing your residence.
- Evacuate to an inland location early if:
  - Local authorities announce an evacuation and you live in an evacuation zone.
  - You live in a mobile home near the path of the hurricane.
  - You live in a high-rise building near the path of the hurricane.
  - You live on the coast, on a flood plain near a river, or on an inland waterway.
  - You feel you are in danger.
- Leave immediately if local authorities order an evacuation. Follow evacuation routes, stay away from coastal areas, riverbanks, and streams, and tell others where you are going.

- If you are not required to evacuate or are unable to evacuate, stay indoors during the hurricane and away from windows and glass doors.
- To protect yourself against strong wind:
  - Take refuge in a small interior room, closet, or hallway.
  - Close all interior doors; secure and brace exterior doors.
  - In a multiple-story building, go to the first or second floors and stay in interior rooms away from windows.
  - Lie on the floor under a table or other sturdy object if a hurricane or any associated tornado approaches.
- Phone lines are likely to be busy with emergency traffic. Avoid using the phone except for serious emergencies.

Landslides

Landslides occur when masses of rock, earth, or debris move down a slope. They occur in almost every US state. Landslides may be small or large and can move at slow or very high speeds. They are usually associated with periods of heavy rainfall or rapid snowmelt.

Safety During a Landslide

Follow these safety guidelines if conditions exist that could cause a landslide:

- Stay alert. Many landslides occur when people are sleeping.
- If you are in areas susceptible to landslides, consider evacuating if it is safe to do so.
- Listen for any unusual sounds that might indicate moving debris, such as trees cracking, boulders knocking together, or rumbling.
- If you are near a stream or channel, be alert for any sudden increase or decrease in water flow and for a change from clear to muddy water. Such changes may indicate landslide activity upstream, so be prepared to move quickly.
- Be alert when driving. Embankments along roadsides are susceptible to landslides. Watch the road for collapsed pavement, mud, fallen rocks, and other indications of possible debris flow.
- In the event that you remain at home, move to a second floor, if possible, to distance yourself from the direct path of landslide debris.

Tornados

A tornado is a violent windstorm characterized by a twisting, funnel-shaped cloud. It is usually spawned by a thun-

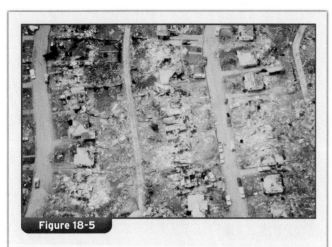

Figure 18-5

The tornado in Wichita Falls, Texas, in 1979 was one of the worst tornadoes in US history.

derstorm or sometimes as a result of a hurricane. Tornado season is generally March through August, although tornadoes can occur at any time of the year. Every state is at some risk from this hazard, but tornados are most frequent east of the Rocky Mountains **Figure 18-5**.

Safety During a Tornado

Follow the following safety guidelines if you experience a tornado.

If you are at home:

- Go immediately to a windowless interior room, storm cellar, basement, or the lowest level of the building. If there is no basement, go to an inner hallway or a smaller inner room without windows, such as a bathroom or closet.
- Get under a piece of sturdy furniture (eg, heavy table or desk) and hold on to it.

If you are outdoors:

- If possible, get inside a building.
- If shelter is not available or there is no time to get indoors, lie in a ditch or low-lying area or crouch near a strong building.

If you are at work or school:

- Avoid places with wide-span roofs, such as auditoriums, cafeterias, large hallways, or shopping malls.
- Go to a predetermined shelter area.
- Get under a piece of sturdy furniture (eg, heavy table, desk, or workbench).

If you are in a vehicle:

- Do not try to out-drive a tornado.
- Get out of the vehicle immediately and take shelter in a nearby building. If there is no time to get indoors, get out of the car and lie in a ditch or low-lying area away from the vehicle.

Tsunamis

A tsunami (pronounced soo-nahm′ee) is a series of waves generated by an undersea disturbance (eg, an earthquake). From the area of disturbance, the waves will travel outward in all directions, much like the ripples caused by throwing a rock into a pond. Tsunamis reaching heights of more than 100 feet have been recorded near coastlines, although most waves are less than 18 feet high. Areas of greatest risk are less than 50 feet above sea level and within 1 mile of the shoreline. Drowning is the most common cause of death.

Safety During a Tsunami

Follow these safety guidelines if conditions exist that could cause a tsunami:

- Listen to a radio or television to get the latest emergency information. If you are advised to evacuate, do so immediately.
- Stay away from the area until local authorities say it is safe.
- Do not go to the shoreline to watch for a tsunami. If you can see the wave, you are too close to escape it. Because a tsunami is a series of waves, do not assume that one wave means that the danger is over.

Volcanic Eruption

A volcano is a mountain that opens downward to a reservoir of molten rock below the earth's surface. When pressure from gases and the molten rock becomes strong enough to cause an explosion, eruptions occur. Gases and rock shoot up through the opening and spill over the mountainsides, and/or spew into the air, filling it with lava fragments and ash.

Safety During a Volcanic Eruption

Follow these safety guidelines in the event of a volcanic eruption:

- Follow the evacuation order issued by local authorities. Avoid areas downwind from the volcano.

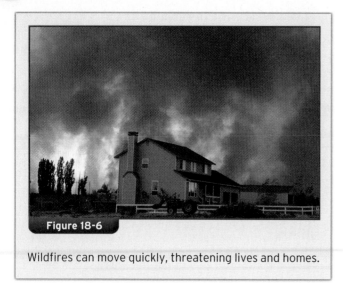

Figure 18-6

Wildfires can move quickly, threatening lives and homes.

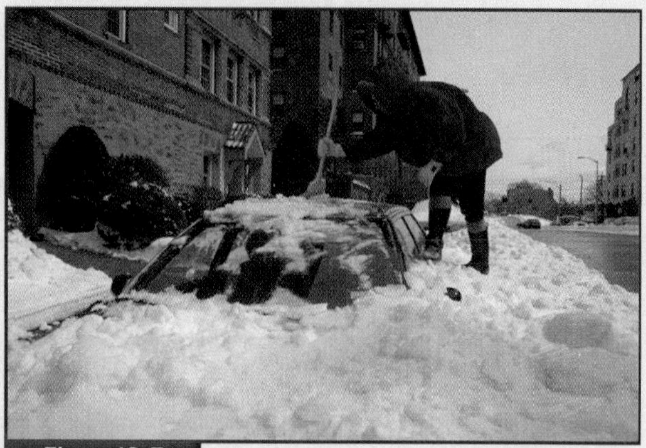

Figure 18-7

Major winter storms can tie up a city.

If caught indoors:
- Close all windows, doors, and chimney and/or stove dampers.
- Put all machinery inside a garage or barn.

If caught outdoors:
- Seek shelter indoors.
- Avoid low-lying areas where poisonous gases can collect and flash floods and mudflows can be dangerous.

Protect yourself:
- Wear long-sleeved shirts and pants.
- Use goggles to protect the eyes.
- Use a dust-mask or hold a damp cloth over your face to help breathing.
- Stay out of the area. Trying to watch an erupting volcano can be deadly.

Wildfires

Forest, brush, and grass fires can occur at any time of the year, but mostly during long, dry hot spells. The majority of these fires are caused by human carelessness or ignorance Figure 18-6 .

Safety During a Wildfire

Follow these safety guidelines in the event of a wildfire:
- Listen to a radio or television to get the latest emergency information.
- If advised to evacuate, do so immediately. Choose a route away from the fire hazard. Watch for changes in the speed and direction of fire and smoke. Do not block firefighting entrance routes.

Winter Storms

Heavy snowfall and extreme cold can immobilize an entire region. Even areas that usually experience mild winters can be hit with a major snowstorm or extreme cold Figure 18-7 .

Safety During a Winter Storm

Adhere to the following safety guidelines in the event of a winter storm:

If indoors:
- Listen to a radio, television, or NOAA Weather Radio for weather reports and emergency information.
- Conserve fuel by lowering the thermostat to 65° F during the day and 55° F at night. Close off unused rooms.
- Eat regularly and drink ample fluids, but avoid caffeine and alcohol.
- If using kerosene heaters, maintain ventilation, refuel the heater outside, and keep heaters at least 3 feet from flammable objects.

If outdoors:
- Dress warmly (eg, several layers of loose fitting clothing, wear a hat, cover mouth with a scarf to protect your lungs).
- Avoid overexertion (eg, shoveling snow or pushing a car), which can bring on a heart attack.
- Be aware of signs of frostbite and hypothermia.
- Keep dry by changing wet clothing, which does not insulate very well.

If trapped in a vehicle during a winter storm:
- Pull off of the highway. Turn on hazard lights. Hang a distress flag from the window or radio antenna.

- Stay inside the vehicle, where rescuers are more likely to find you. Do not set out on foot unless you can see a building close by where you know you can take shelter.
- Run the engine and heater about 10 minutes each hour to keep warm. When the engine is running, open a window slightly for ventilation and clear snow from the exhaust pipe to protect against carbon monoxide poisoning.
- Exercise (eg, clap hands and move arms and legs occasionally) to maintain body heat, but avoid overexertion.
- In extreme cold, use floor mats, seat covers, road maps, newspapers, and other available resources for insulation. Huddle with other passengers.
- Take turns sleeping. One person should be awake at all times to look for rescue crews.
- Drink fluids to avoid dehydration.
- Watch for signs of frostbite and hypothermia.
- Be careful not to waste battery power.
- At night, turn on the inside light so work crews or rescuers can see you.
- Once the winter storm passes, you may need to leave the car and proceed on foot.

FYI

Winter Travel Supplies

When traveling during the winter, carry disaster supplies in the vehicle. The kit should include the following:

- Shovel
- Windshield scraper
- Flashlight
- Extra batteries
- Battery-powered radio
- Water
- Snack food
- Gloves and mittens
- Hat
- Blanket
- Tow chain or rope
- Tire chains
- Bag of road salt and sand
- Fluorescent distress flag
- Jumper or booster cables
- Road maps
- Emergency flares
- Cellular telephone

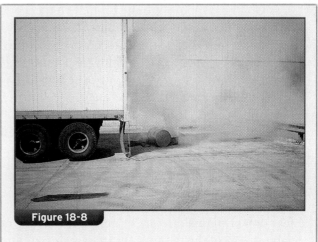

Figure 18-8

Fumes leaking from a cargo truck could be an indication of a hazardous materials incident.

▶ Technological Hazards

Hazardous Materials Incidents

Chemicals are found everywhere. They can become hazardous during their production, storage, transportation, or disposal. It is not always possible to identify a situation as one involving hazardous materials, but clues such as a leaking cargo trailer, color-coded placards (signs) on abandoned drums, and unusual odors are good indicators **Figure 18-8**.

Safety During a Hazardous Materials Incident

Follow these safety guidelines in the event of a hazardous materials incident:

- If you witness an incident that you believe to a hazardous materials incident, call 9-1-1 or your local emergency telephone number.
- Stay away from the incident site.
- If caught outside, remember that gases and mists are usually heavier than air. Try to stay upstream, uphill, and upwind. Try to go at least one-half mile from the danger area.
- If in a vehicle, stop and seek shelter in a building, if possible. If you must remain in the vehicle, keep windows and vents closed and shut off the air conditioner and heater.
- If asked to evacuate your home, do so immediately.
- If requested to stay indoors rather than evacuate:
  - Follow all instructions; close all exterior doors, windows, vents, and fireplace dampers.
  - Turn off air conditioners and ventilation systems.

- Go into an above-ground room with the fewest openings to the outside; close doors and windows; tape around the sides, bottom, and top of the door; cover each window and vent in the room with a single piece of plastic sheeting.
- Listen to emergency broadcasts.
- When advised to leave your shelter, open all doors and windows and turn on air conditioning and ventilation systems to flush out any chemicals that infiltrated the building.

Nuclear Power Plants

Nuclear power plants operate in most states and produce about 20% of the nation's power. Nearly 3 million Americans live within 10 miles of an operating nuclear power plant. Although these plants are monitored and regulated closely, unintentional radiation exposures are possible. Local and state governments, federal agencies, and the electric utilities have emergency response plans in the event of a nuclear power plant incident.

Safety During a Nuclear Power Plant Emergency

Follow these safety guidelines in the event of a nuclear power plant emergency:

- Stay tuned to local radio and television. Local authorities will provide specific information and instructions.
- Evacuate if you are advised to do so.
- If told not to evacuate, remain indoors. Close doors and windows, and turn off the air conditioner, ventilation fans, furnace, and other air intakes. Go to a basement or other underground area if possible. Keep a battery-powered radio with you at all times.
- Do not use the telephone unless absolutely necessary. Lines will be needed for emergency calls.
- If you suspect exposure, take a thorough shower. Change clothes and shoes. Put exposed clothing in a plastic bag. Seal the bag and place it out of the way.
- Seek medical care for any unusual symptoms, like nausea, which may be related to radiation exposure.

▶ National Security Emergencies

Terrorism

Terrorism is the use of force or violence against persons or property in violation of the criminal laws of the United States for purposes of intimidation, coercion, or ransom. Acts of terrorism range from threats of terrorism, assassinations, kidnappings, hijackings, bomb scares and bombings, and cyber attacks (computer-based attacks), to the use of chemical, biologic, and nuclear weapons (Figure 18-9).

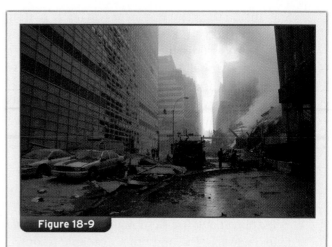

Figure 18-9

The September 11, 2001, terrorist attack on the World Trade Center in New York City.

Table 18-1	Homeland Security Advisory System
Threat Level	**Protective Measures You Should Take**
Severe	Avoid high-risk areas such as public gatherings.
	Listen attentively to news for advisories and instructions.
	Contact employers to determine work status.
High	Review evacuation and sheltering measures for different types of attacks (chemical, biologic, or radiologic).
Elevated	Watch and report any suspicious activity. Contact school(s) to determine their emergency procedures.
Guarded	Review home disaster plan and update supplies.
	Meet with your family to discuss what to do, where to go, and how to communicate if an attack occurs.
Low	Develop a home disaster plan and disaster supply kit.

The Homeland Security Advisory System is designed to provide quick, comprehensive information concerning the potential threat of terrorist attacks or threat levels. Threat conditions can apply nationally, regionally, by industry, or by specific target. You should be aware of the current Homeland Security Threat Level at all times (Table 18-1).

Chemical and Biologic Agents

<u>Chemical warfare agents</u> are poisonous vapors, aerosols, liquids, or solids that have toxic effects on people, animals, or plants. They can be released by bombs; sprayed from aircraft, boats, or vehicles; or used as a liquid to create a hazard to people and the environment. Some chemical agents are odorless and tasteless. They can have an immediate effect (a few seconds to a few minutes) or a delayed effect (several hours to several days). Although potentially lethal, chemical agents are difficult to deliver in lethal concentrations. When released outdoors, the agents often dissipate rapidly.

<u>Biologic agents</u> are organisms or toxins that can kill or incapacitate people, livestock, or crops. The three basic groups of biologic agents likely to be used as weapons are bacteria, viruses, and toxins.

Safety During a Chemical or Biologic Attack

In the case of a chemical or biologic weapon attack, authorities will instruct you on the best course of action. This may be to evacuate the area immediately, to seek shelter at a designated location, or to take immediate shelter where you are and seal the premises. The best way to protect yourself is to take emergency preparedness measures ahead of time and to get medical attention as soon as possible, if needed.

Follow these additional safety guidelines in the event of a chemical or biologic attack:

- Listen to a radio or television for instructions from authorities, such as whether to remain inside or to evacuate.
- If instructed to remain in your home, office building, or other shelter during a chemical or biologic attack:
  - Turn off all ventilation, including furnaces, air conditioners, vents, and fans.
  - Seek shelter in an internal room, preferably one without windows. Seal the room with duct tape and plastic sheeting.
  - Avoid the furnace or utility room.
  - Do not use any major appliances (eg, furnace, oven/range, clothes dryer, or washing machine).
- Remain in protected areas where toxic vapors are reduced or eliminated, and be sure to take a battery-operated radio with you.
- If caught in an unprotected area: Try to get upwind of the contaminated area, find shelter inside a building as quickly as possible, and listen to the radio for official instructions.

Nuclear and Radiologic Weapons

Nuclear explosions can cause deadly effects, such as blinding light, intense heat (thermal radiation), initial nuclear radiation, blast fires started by the heat pulse, and secondary fires caused by the destruction. Above ground explosions also produce radioactive particles called *fallout* that can be carried by wind for hundreds of miles.

Terrorist use of a radiologic dispersion device (RDD)—often called a "dirty bomb"—is considered far more likely than the use of a nuclear device. Such radiologic weapons are a combination of conventional explosives and radioactive material designed to scatter dangerous and sublethal amounts of radioactive material over a general area.

There is no way of knowing how much warning time there would be before an attack by a terrorist using a nuclear or radiologic weapon.

Safety During a Nuclear or Radiologic Attack

Follow these safety guidelines in the event of a nuclear or radiologic attack:

- Avoid looking at the flash or fireball—it can blind you.
- If you hear an attack warning:
  - Take cover as quickly as you can, below ground if possible, and stay there unless instructed to do otherwise.
  - If caught outside and unable to get inside immediately, take cover behind anything that might offer protection. Lie flat on the ground and cover your head.
  - If the explosion is some distance away, it could take 30 seconds or more for the blast wave to hit. Be aware of a second, returning blast wave.
- Protect yourself from radioactive fallout by taking shelter, even if you are many miles from the source of the explosion.
- Keep a battery-powered radio with you, and listen for official information. Follow the instructions given. Local instructions should always take precedence: Officials in your area know the local situation best.

▶ Summary

"The farther you are from the last disaster, the closer you are to the next one" is an often quoted statement made by emergency preparedness specialists. We live in an age of catastrophe. Every American will likely be an unfortunate victim or witness to at least one disaster during his or her lifetime.

The tragedy of disasters is that we can all be better prepared than we are now. When a disaster strikes, you must be ready to act.

FYI

Disaster Preparedness

The US Department of Homeland Security offers these general guidelines for food and water needs for survival during emergency situations:

Water

- One gallon of water per person per day, for drinking and sanitation.
- Children, nursing mothers, and people who are ill may need more water.
- If you live in a warm climate, more water may be necessary.
- Keep at least a 3-day supply of water per person.

Food

- Store at least a 3-day supply of nonperishable food.
- Select foods that require no refrigeration, preparation, or cooking and little or no water.
- Pack a manual can opener and eating utensils.
- Choose foods your family will eat:
    - Ready-to-eat canned meats, fruits, and vegetables
    - Protein or fruit bars
    - Dry cereal or granola
    - Peanut butter
    - Dried fruit
    - Nuts
    - Crackers
    - Canned juices
    - Nonperishable pasteurized milk
    - High-energy foods
    - Vitamins
    - Food for infants
    - Comfort foods

▶ Ready for Review

- Disaster is a fact of life, and you need to be prepared.
- The farther you are from the last disaster, the closer you are to the next one.
- Natural disasters such as earthquakes, floods, hurricanes, and tornadoes claim many lives each year. Being informed about their dangers protects you and others and can help minimize injuries and deaths.
- Chemicals are found everywhere. It is not always possible to identify a situation as one involving hazardous materials, but clues such as leaking cargo trailers, placards or signs on abandoned drums, and unusual odors can be good indicators.
- Terrorism is the use of force or violence against persons or property in violation of the criminal laws of the United States for purposes of intimidation, coercion, or ransom.

▶ Vital Vocabulary

biologic agents Organisms or toxins that can kill or incapacitate people, livestock, or crops.

chemical warfare agents Poisonous vapors, aerosols, liquids, or solids that have toxic effects.

terrorism Use of force or violence against persons of property in violation of criminal laws for purposes of intimidation, coercion, or ransom.

tsunami A series of waves generated by an undersea disturbance.

▶ Assessment in Action

It is early September, and you are visiting your retired grandparents at their ocean-front home on the Gulf Coast. While listening to the television, you learn that a hurricane is heading your way within the next 24 hours.

Directions: Circle *Yes* if you agree with the statement and *No* if you disagree.

Yes No 1. You should board up the windows to prevent the risk of broken glass.

Yes No 2. Don't take the time to fill up your car with gas, because there are plenty of gasoline stations along the highway.

Yes No 3. Review all possible evacuation routes before driving.

Yes No 4. Take any medications that you or your grandparents use.

Yes No 5. Be on the lookout for tornadoes.

Answers: 1. Yes; 2. No; 3. Yes; 4. Yes; 5. Yes

▶ Check Your Knowledge

Directions: Circle *Yes* if you agree with the statement and *No* if you disagree.

Yes No 1. Earthquakes occur most often in the winter.

Yes No 2. Never drive or walk through moving flood water.

Yes No 3. People in urban areas may be at greater risk from the effects of a prolonged heat wave than those in rural areas.

Yes No 4. Hurricane season is from April until August.

Yes No 5. Seek shelter in a room with open windows if you are in the path of a tornado.

Yes No 6. Never go near the shoreline to watch for a tsunami.

Yes No 7. If you experience a tornado alert, go to a shopping mall, school auditorium, or cafeteria.

Yes No 8. To survive during emergency situations, the average person should have 1 gallon of water for drinking and sanitation each day.

Yes No 9. If you are caught in your car during a blizzard, you should keep your engine running at all times and the car windows rolled up to prevent hypothermia.

Yes No 10. If you are caught outside during a tornado, seek cover in a low-lying area, such as a ditch.

Answers: 1. No; 2. Yes; 3. Yes; 4. No; 5. No; 6. Yes; 7. No; 8. Yes; 9. No; 10. Yes

index

Chapter 1

Opener Courtesy of Lawrence Newell; 1–1 Reproduced from U.S. Department of Labor, Bureau of Labor Statistics: Sprains and strains most common workplace injury. Monthly Labor Review, April 1, 2005. Available at: http://www.bls.gov/opub/ted/2005/mar/wk4/art05.htm.; 1–2 Vyrostek SB, Annest JL, Ryan GW. Surveillance for Fatal and Nonfatal Injuries— United States, 2001. MMWR 53(SSO7);1–75 (September 3, 2004); 1–3 Courtesy of Ellis and Associates.

Chapter 2

Opener © Peter Steiner/Alamy Images.

Chapter 3

Opener © Ingram Publishing/age fotostock; 3–2 © Jonathan Noden-Wilkinson/ShutterStock, Inc.; 3–5 Courtesy of MedicAlert Foundation®. © 2006, All Rights Reserved. MedicAlert® is a federally registered trademark and service mark.

Chapter 4

Opener Courtesy of Lawrence Newell; 4–5 Photographed by Kimberly Potvin.

Chapter 5

Opener Courtesy of Lawrence Newell; 5–2 Source: American Heart Association; 5–9 Courtesy of Phillips Medical Systems. All rights reserved.

Chapter 6

Opener © Jones and Bartlett Publishers. Photographed by Christine McKeen.; 6–5 © Howard Backer.

Chapter 7

Opener © Jones and Bartlett Publishers. Photographed by Christine McKeen.; 7–4 Courtesy of Dey, L.P.

Chapter 9

Opener © Joe Gough/ShutterStock, Inc.

Chapter 10

Opener © Gordon Swanson/ShutterStock, Inc.

Chapter 11

Opener © Christoph & Friends/Das Fotoarchiv./Alamy Images.

Chapter 12

Opener © Jones and Bartlett Publishers. Courtesy of MIEMSS.

Chapter 13

Opener © Stockbyte/Creatas; 13–4 A: © Thomas Photography LLC/Alamy Images; 13–4 B: © Thomas J. Peterson/Alamy Images; 13–4 C: Courtesy of US Fish & Wildlife Service.

Chapter 14

Opener © Jonathan Plant/Alamy Images; 14–3 © AbleStock; 14–4 Courtesy of Ray Rauch/U.S. Fish & Wildlife Services; 14–5 Courtesy of South Florida Water Management District; 14–6 Courtesy of Luther C. Goldman/U.S. Fish & Wildlife Service; 14–10 A: © Borut Gorenjak/ShutterStock, Inc.; 14–10 B: © Dwight Lyman/ShutterStock, Inc.; 14–10 C: © pixelman/ShutterStock, Inc.; 14–10 D: © Heintje Joseph T. Lee/ShutterStock, Inc.; 14–13 © photobar/ShutterStock, Inc.; 14–14 Courtesy of Kenneth Cramer, Monmouth College; 14–16 © Nick Simon/ShutterStock, Inc.; 14–17 © Kirubeshwaran/ShutterStock, Inc.

Chapter 15

Opener © Maxim Petrichuk/ShutterStock, Inc.; FYI box on page 167, Courtesy of the National Weather Service/NOAA.

Chapter 16

Opener © Laura Rauch/AP Photos.

Chapter 17

17–3 © U.S. Department of Transportation.; 17–4 © U.S. Department of Transportation.

Chapter 18

Opener Courtesy of Dave Saville/FEMA; 18–1 Courtesy of D. Perkins/USGS; 18–2 Courtesy of Jocelyn Augustino/FEMA; 18–4 © Photos.com; 18–5 Courtesy of the National Weather Service Forecast Office/NOAA; 18–6 Courtesy of John Hutmacher/USFS; 18–7 © Ron Frehm/AP Photos; 18–9 Courtesy of Andrea Booher/FEMA.

Notes

Notes

Notes

Notes

Notes